Praise for *Your Hidden Food Allergies Are Making You Fat*

"I have seen the ALCAT test work and produce tremendous beneficial results."

—DAVID L. CROOKS, M.D.,
instructor of genetics and immunology,
Stanford University School of Medicine

"The ALCAT test is revolutionary! It is a must for doctors who wish to offer the best allergy test to their patients. It has changed the way I practice."

—MIKELL SUZANNE PARSONS, DC, CCN, DACBN
Assistant Professor of Clinical Sciences,
University of Bridgeport

"I've seen the [ALCAT] technique work when absolutely no other approach has made the scale budge."

—STEVEN LAMM, M.D.,
author of *Thinner at Last*

"98 percent of the subjects following the ALCAT plan either lost weight or improved body composition."

—from a study at Baylor Sports Medicine
and Performance Institute

Your Hidden Food Allergies Are Making You Fat, Revised

For more information on the ALCAT test, please contact

Cell Science Systems, Corp.
852 South Military Trail
Deerfield Beach, FL 33442 USA
Tel.: (954) 426-2304
www.ALCAT.com

In Europe:
Alcat Europe, GmbH
Bio Tech Park
Neuendorfstrasse 24b
16761 Hennigsdorf
Germany
Tel.: +49 3302 2023800
www.ALCAT-Europe.com

Your Hidden Food Allergies Are Making You Fat, Revised

**RUDY RIVERA, M.D., AND
ROGER DAVIS DEUTSCH**

THREE RIVERS PRESS • NEW YORK

Library of Congress Cataloging-in-Publication Data
Rivera, Rudy.
    Your hidden food allergies are making you fat, revised : how to lose weight
and gain years of vitality / Rudy Rivera, Roger Deutsch.
        Includes bibliographical references and index.
        1. Food allergy—Complications. 2. Weight loss. 3. Obesity—Etiology.
    4. Blood—Examination. I. Deutsch, Roger. II. Title.
    RC596.D485 2002
    616.97'5—dc21   2002070522

ISBN 0-7615-3760-0

15 14 13 12 11

Printed in the United States of America

Second Edition

*Dedicated to my loving wife
whose memory keeps me dreaming against all odds.
And to my two sons and daughter
who gave up their time with me
so this book could be written.*

—RUDY RIVERA

*This book is dedicated to the spirit of all those who
seek to uplift the well-being of all humanity without
seeking personal reward, and to my family.*

—ROGER DAVIS DEUTSCH

CONTENTS

Foreword by Dr. David M. Brady　xi

Preface　xiii

Introduction　xv

1　A Medical Breakthrough for the 21st Century　1

2　Overweight: The Plague of Our Age　27

3　Breakthrough Research on Obesity and Health　62

4　A Short Course in the Science of Food Intolerance　85

5　Overweight: As American As Apple Pie　110

6　Yo-Yo Dieting　138

7　Food Intolerance: The Missed Diagnosis　158

8　Food Sensitivities and Overweight　176

9　The Right Diet for the 21st Century　194

10　Airways and Food Intolerance　226

11　Skin and Food Intolerance　238

12   Fatigue and Food Intolerance   254

13   Migraine and Food Intolerance   271

14   Food Intolerance: How to Live With It   288

Bibliography of Selected ALCAT Test Studies   309

Index   315

About the Authors   329

FOREWORD

In my many years of teaching and practicing nutritional and integrative medicine, I have had the opportunity to investigate and apply a plethora of conventional and alternative laboratory tests for a broad spectrum of diverse and complicated patient conditions.

The right test for the right patient can provide both the clinician and patient with valuable insight into the patient's situation, and thus determine and then monitor the progress of an individually designed therapeutic intervention.

Amongst all of these laboratory tests, I have found the ALCAT test to be one of the most valuable in getting to the bottom of most of the problems that cause a patient to seek the help of either an alternative or conventional doctor. As is seen from the many clinical research studies and case histories presented in this book, the ALCAT test has helped in a multitude of chronic cases where other investigations and treatments had reached a dead end.

In this time of increasing rates of obesity, diabetes, cardiovascular disease, autoimmune diseases, and many other difficult-to-explain degenerative disorders in patients of all ages, understanding and then utilizing the ALCAT test, I am convinced, will provide a profound and lasting benefit to individuals and to our health care system at large.

The authors have performed a brilliant job of explaining the nature of food and chemical intolerance, and how this unique and practical medical breakthrough test can identify such occurrences, leading to weight loss, increased vitality, and overall wellness. They have done so in clear and simple terms, yet with sufficient breadth and scope that this book will be of immense interest to both health professionals and the health-conscious layman alike.

They put forward a clear and concise picture of the many elements of nutritional, biochemical, genetic and sociological theory, unified into a coherent, easy to understand principle of approaching health issues on the basis of each individual's unique relationship to his or her environment and diet.

I am certain that this book will find its place among the many classic books on health, such as Dr. Roger Williams' *Biochemical Individuality,* which is still studied nearly fifty years after its first publication, and that this book will provide meaningful answers to current dilemmas and exert a positive influence on the way we view the many new health challenges confronting modern industrial society.

Dr. David M. Brady
Chair, Department of Clinical Sciences
University of Bridgeport
Bridgeport, Connecticut (USA)

PREFACE

The aim of this book is to bring about awareness of the true cause of the current crisis in health care and at the same time offer a realistic and practical solution to both the individual and societal health problems common today. The goal is to minimize the high incidence of obesity and all the degenerative diseases associated with the aging process. The solution we propose is a fundamental change in the approach to preventing the diseases of modern life. It is based on a breakthrough medical technology, a simple blood test that is capable of identifying an individual's genetically determined, immune system response to dietary and other environmental factors.

When this book was first released in late 1998, a clinical study from Baylor Medical College had recently been published in the *Journal of the American Society of Bariatric Medicine*. It reported that 98 percent of the subjects who had treatment based on the ALCAT test had success either losing weight and/or improvement in body composition during a one-month study. This finding followed a decade of reports from physicians using the ALCAT test around the world who claimed that their patients were losing weight, that the weight loss predominantly consisted of adipose tissue, and that this achievement was effortless, without caloric restriction, and was maintained for as long as the patient continued to follow the guidelines based on his or her test results.

The book came out at a time when the medical profession, the media, and therefore the public, had a fascination with weight loss drugs, which the FDA (Food and Drug Administration) has since removed from the market because of their dangerous and sometimes fatal side effects. We believe drugs are not necessary in most cases to lose weight or to treat other diseases characteristic of modern industrial society, such as migraine, irritable bowel syndrome, hyperactivity and attention deficit, fatigue, depression, and many others. Dietary modification based on scientific assessment of an individual's genetically based immune system susceptibilities is usually sufficient.

This updated version of *Your Hidden Food Allergies Are Making You Fat: How to Lose Weight and Gain Years of Vitality* explains the research and other findings that have come to light over the past few years that convincingly demonstrate how the appropriate use of this breakthrough technology can restore effectiveness to our ailing health care system and help individuals live longer and healthier lives.

INTRODUCTION

A New Scenario

The past century has brought tremendous changes to our social health condition. By developing antibiotics, vaccinations, and improvements in public hygiene, medical science and technology have eliminated a substantial number of infectious diseases. But other consequences of technological development have created new and ever more complicated health problems.

On the positive side, more of Earth's burgeoning population in industrialized societies is being fed because commercialized agriculture has significantly increased volume yields. Life expectancy has increased markedly in most countries since the beginning of the 20th century. As Sir Robert May, current president of the Royal Society (the United Kingdom's National Academy of Science, founded in 1660) and former Chief Scientific Advisor to Her Majesty's Government puts it, "Today, worldwide, most people live longer and are better fed than ever before." He goes on to say, "These benefits, however, have environmental and other costs."

It is these "environmental costs" that are responsible for the dramatic decline in our health. The technological development that has increased life expectancy is a double-edged sword. Whereas infectious diseases have been reduced substantially, chronic degenerative disorders, such as obesity, cancers, heart conditions, diabetes, and several less-defined problems, such as fatigue and cognitive impairment, are increasing at alarming rates.

Even though we now enjoy a greater life expectancy at the time of birth, the increase in life span of those who made it through childhood has not been all that significant. A 50-year-old in 1900 could expect to live an additional 21.3 years. In 1998 the average 50-year-old can anticipate 29.8 more years of survival. The marked difference in improvement in life expectancy versus life span is because, in 1900, 13 percent of children in the United States died before their first birthday. Today, given better prevention and treatment of infectious disease, that number is less than 1 percent.

To gain further insight into the nature of the current health challenges, one need only look at the major causes of death over the past 100 years. In the United States in 1900, cancer was responsible for only 3.3 percent of deaths. Today the number has risen to 25 percent. Heart disease killed 14.2 percent in 1900. Today, heart disease is responsible for 33 percent of deaths. Looking at the causes of death in Chile for the same time frame, in the earlier period almost half of all deaths, 46.6 percent, resulted from various infectious diseases, whereas a relatively small number of deaths, 14.8 percent, were attributable to cancers and cardiovascular disease. However, by 1999 the situation had dramatically changed. Deaths caused by infectious disease had dropped to 20.9 percent, whereas those from cancers and cardiovascular diseases had soared to 53.2 percent. This statistical pattern is typical of industrialized societies and reflects the impact of environmental changes occurring during the past century.

Although a number of experts believe the increase of life span itself accounts for these degenerative diseases, in several cultures where the life span is as great or even greater than that of the United States, the incidence of such disorders is considerably less. Coincidentally, these cultures have maintained the native diet to a great extent. Such is the case in Japan, France, and several Mediterranean countries. There are also reports of average life spans of 120 years among the Hunzas of eastern Pakistan, as well as among the Vilkabaumba Indians and Titacacas of South America, and others, where the impact of technology is virtually absent.

The United States is the world's most technologically advanced country and also spends the most on health care, about 15 percent of the gross national product (GNP), or approximately $1 trillion per year. Yet its citizens do not enjoy the longest life expectancy, nor does it have the lowest incidence of cancer, heart disease, obesity, or diabetes.

In fact, the United States is the world leader among major countries in the prevalence of weight problems, estimated at 67 percent of all adults. Only the inhabitants of a small South Pacific country (Samoa) exceed Americans' rate of obesity. American children are also fatter now than at any time before. According to a study reported in *JAMA* (*Journal of the American Medical Association*) in December 2001, by Dr. Richard Strauss of the Robert Wood Johnson Medical School and Harold Pollack of the University of Michigan, 22 percent of African-American and Hispanic kids, and 12 percent of Caucasian kids, aged 4 to 12, are overweight. This represents an alarming increase of more than 50 percent over the previous 12 years.

More than 16 million Americans also suffer from diabetes, and 10 million more are at high risk of developing it.

Of these cases, 95 percent are of the adult onset type. In this form of the disease, the islet cells of the pancreas produce too little insulin, or the muscle cells that require insulin to transport glucose inside them, so that it can be converted to energy, become insensitive to the insulin that is produced. Both causes are related to overweight and immune dysfunction. Diabetes and obesity are so interlinked that Dr. David Heber, head of the UCLA Center for Human Nutrition, refers to the combined syndrome as "diabesity." The cost to the U.S. health care system for treating diabetes exceeds $100 billion per year.

Looking at these statistics, one can't avoid the conclusion that various lifestyle factors, particularly dietary habits, play a major role in the incidence of such disorders. That's not new. It is new, however, that the profundity of its impact is now appreciated and that the technology for determining the best possible diet for any given individual is now available in the form of a breakthrough laboratory test. This test determines an individual's specific, genetically based, immune system response to dietary factors, as well as to chemicals, drugs, and other substances.

Health Management or Disease Management?

Considering the money spent on health care, in relationship to the societal degree of health, to refer to the American medical system as a *"health* care" system is really a misnomer. Rather, it is a *disease management* system. It is designed to cope with the effect of technology's impact on agriculture and society, which has replaced many old diseases with new ones. The more obvious of these include not only obesity, cardiovascular disease, diabetes, and cancer, as already discussed, but also chronic fatigue, various autoimmune disorders, including arthritis, mental conditions (such as depression and attention deficit hyperactivity disorder, or ADHD), migraine, and others. These problems are primarily caused by the food we eat, high levels of environmental pollution, a general lack of exercise, and other lifestyle factors. Thus, with the right emphasis on prevention, most of these problems can be avoided.

In addition to the increased challenges posed by a more polluted environment, we must also contend with the many deficiencies created by a less nutritious food supply. As part of a doctoral thesis at Johns Hopkins University, Virginia Worthington reviewed 41 studies comparing the nutritional value of commercially grown versus organic foods. She reports that before World War II, agricultural chemicals were virtually nonexistent. However, by 1995 commercial agricultural practices in the United States consumed 45 million tons of artificial fertilizers and 770 million pounds of poisonous pesticides each year, equaling nearly 3 pounds of pesticide for every American man, woman, and child. In 1999, approximately 95 percent of all produced crops used these chemicals.

The explosion of chemical use in agriculture after World War II occurred because the Germans and the Americans needed a place to dump all their surplus stores of poisonous chemicals left over from the war. They determined that with the right marketing spin, dumping them into our agricultural system food supply would provide them with the most economic gain.

In her report, "Nutritional Quality of Organic Versus Conventional Fruits, Vegetables and Grains" (*Journal of Alternative and Complementary Medicine,* vol. 7, issue 2, November 2001), Worthington states, "Organic crops contained significantly more vitamin C, iron, magnesium, and phosphorus and significantly less nitrates than conventional crops. There were non-significant trends showing less protein but of a better quality and a higher content of nutritionally significant minerals with lower amounts of some heavy metals in organic crops. There appear to be genuine differences in the nutrient content of organic and conventional crops."

As nutritional quantity and quality decline in our food intake, so does our ability to detoxify foreign chemicals and neutralize free radicals because these processes require vitamins, minerals, and protein from our diet. We are further impaired in our ability to perform basic biological functions, such as tissue repair, energy metabolism, and protein synthesis. Against this backdrop, the many pollution exposures we face will induce overactivation of the immune system, thus depleting immune resources and rendering us prone to premature aging, obesity, diabetes, frequent infections, and chronic degenerative disease, including cancer.

If that were not enough, we now have yet another "technological breakthrough" affecting our food supply to cope with. Genetically modified (GM) foods that entered the marketplace in 1996 are now contained in an estimated 60 to 70 percent of all processed foods. The U.S. FDA comments, "Genetic engineering may transfer new and unidentified proteins from one food to another, triggering allergic reactions. Millions of Americans who are sensitive to allergens will have no way of identifying or protecting themselves from offending foods" (*Fed I Register 22987- Federal Register,* Vol. 57, number 104, May 29, 1992).

Studies documenting the adverse health effects of genetically modified foods are already surfacing. GM soybeans contain higher levels of known allergy provokers. In lab studies, rats suffer immune system, thymus, kidney, spleen, and intestinal damage from eating GM potatoes, according to Dr. Arpad Pusztai from the Rowett Institute in Scotland. Resistance to antibiotics is yet another concern. Dr. John Fagan, who conducted research for the National Institutes of Health, believes more research should be conducted before GM foods are available. Many others agree, yet once again commercial interests have prevailed. Reports of the health effects from environmental pollution are also increasing. Researchers from England, led by Martine Vrijheid, Ph.D., from the London School of Hygiene and Tropical Medicine, reported in the January 26, 2002, issue of *The Lancet,* that the risk of nongenetic birth defects is one third greater among people living within 2 miles of 21 toxic waste dumps in Europe than among people living between 2 and 4 miles from such sites.

In another recent study, a team from UCLA reported in the December 29, 2001, issue of the *American Journal of Epidemiology* that the likelihood of heart defects at birth can be increased as much as 300 percent for people living near freeways. According to Dr. Beate Ritz, lead investigator, "The greater a woman's exposure to one of these two pollutants (ozone and carbon monoxide) in the critical second month of pregnancy, the greater the chance that her child will have one of these serious cardiac birth defects."

Understanding Brings Hope

However, in the midst of this dilemma it appears that medical science may be on the verge of understanding the modern plague of cardiovascular disease, obesity, and diabetes. Dr. Bruce Bartholomew Duncan and Dr. Maria Ines Schmidt, of the Federal University do Rio Grande do Sul, in Brazil, recently reported that the cluster of disorders referred to by the World Health Organization as metabolic syndrome—which includes cardiovascular disease, obesity and diabetes—is probably caused by chronic activation of the innate immune system (Chronic activation of the innate immune system may underlie the metabolic syndrome, *Sao Paulo Medical Journal,* May 2001 vol. 119, no. 3).

The work done by these authors represents a major breakthrough in understanding this modern plague.

It has become clear, as Duncan and Schmidt explain in their review, that well-known biomarkers of inflammation interlink these conditions and that they all stem from overactivity of the innate immune system. The innate immune system, as distinguished from the adaptive or specific immune system, as explained in more detail later, is the first to engage against assaults from various pathogens, trauma, and stress. Our research over the past 17 years, involving many different clinical and research sites, has looked at the relationship between the exposure to foreign substances and a wide range of clinical symptoms. The test marker that we are looking for is activation of the immune system, particularly, the innate immune system. These studies, which are described in this book, have clearly demonstrated that incompatible foods, food additives, chemicals, and environmental insults are major factors that chronically activate the innate immune system, thus giving rise to metabolic syndrome. In one study carried out in the UK and reported at the 45th Annual Congress of the American College of Allergy & Immunology, Nov. 12–16, 1988, the investigators, Drs. Peter J. Fell and Jonathan Brostoff from England, found an 83.4 percent correlation with ALCAT test results and double-blind oral challenge tests with foods. A study from Copenhagen performed by Dr. Lene Høj, presented at the 52nd annual meeting of the American Academy of Allergy, Asthma & Immunology in January of 1996, reported a 96 percent correlation with double-blind placebo controlled oral challenges with food additives. A study conducted at Baylor Medical College , also reported in 1996 in the spring issue of the medical weight loss journal *The Bariatrician,* determined 98 percent success with weight loss and/or improvement in body composition.

The effects of this metabolic syndrome are far reaching and include disturbance to potentially any organ or bodily system. It can also suppress vitally important sex hormones such as estrogen, testosterone, and growth hormone. When these hormones are in balance and at healthy levels, they protect against diseases of aging and contribute to well-being on all levels. Declining levels are associated with aging and degeneration. Replenishing hormones to more youthful levels, using synthetic and even "bioidentical" hormones, creates the risk of hormone imbalance and other metabolic consequences. Thus preventing damage to the endocrine system and preventing the generation of stress hormones, which are associated with metabolic syndrome, represent a preferred and now available option.

Duncan and Schmidt's paper provides a critical link to the understanding of how best to address these problems. The authors conclude, "Better understanding of the role of the innate immune system in the pathophysiology of obesity, diabetes, the metabolic syndrome, and cardiovascular disease as well as of the causes of chronic activation of this system may lead to important advances in the prediction and management of these chronic diseases." The ALCAT test, which has been the object of our study for many years, does provide a clear understanding of the role of the innate immune system in this disease process and is probably the most important step toward solving the problem.

In this book we explain this scientific, inexpensive, and convenient laboratory blood test, which rapidly identifies any individual's unique reactions to commonly encountered foods, additives, environmental chemicals, molds, common drugs, herbs, and other substances that cause biochemical imbalance. We believe these are the *main* triggers causing the inappropriate and chronic activation of the innate immune system described by Drs. Duncan and Schmidt. Avoiding substances indicated by the test reverses many disease conditions, restoring health, normal weight, and well-being.

The profound benefit of such intervention is illustrated by an outcome study recently reported by a private clinic in Copenhagen that documents significant benefits through application of the ALCAT test in a real-life clinical practice.

An Ancient Perspective

The concept, however, is certainly not new. Hippocrates, the father of modern medicine, although born about 2,500 years ago, on the Greek island of Cos, continues to exert a strong influence on the theoretical practice of modern medicine. The oath he created for doctors is recited by nearly all newly trained physicians at the time of their graduation from medical school. Hippocrates is also known to have said,

> [It] appears to me necessary to every physician to be skilled in nature, and to strive to know, if he would wish to perform his duties, what man is in relation to the articles of food and drink, and to his occupations, and what are the effects of each of them to everyone.

A similar admonition is echoed by Lucretius, another of the renowned ancient physicians: "Let thy food be thy medicine and thy medicine be thy food."

A crucial part of the Hippocratic oath is "First, do no harm." Yet an estimated 140,000 deaths occur each year in the United States as a direct result of adverse drug reactions. The technological culture and disease management paradigm, driven by economic interests, has created a system where we take "a pill for every ill" and "a drug for every bug" and ignores this fundamental measure of disease prevention and health preservation.

To be sure, the current medical paradigm reflects the character of modern industrial life: fast food, fast pace, and less contact with nature. Nonetheless, even though our lifestyles have changed dramatically over the past five or so generations, our genetic makeup has not. Dr. Loren Cordain, author of *The Paleo Diet* (2002), reckons that the human genome is 99.98 percent the same as it was 40,000 years ago. We are Stone Age organisms living in an altered and artificial environment to which we have not adapted. And the more artificial the environment becomes, which most definitely includes our food, the less able we are to adapt to it, and the sicker we become.

In the last 100 years disease prevention and health preservation has been relegated to an inferior state amid the excitement generated by the truly amazing scientific and technological breakthroughs in the areas of diagnostics and imaging, drug therapeutics, as well better understanding of the human genome. The mapping of the human genome opens the potential of using gene therapy to treat many inherited disorders. Such discoveries have brought many benefits, but they have also split our health care system into two fairly distinct branches.

The mainstream branch embraces the application of scientific reductionist principles to treat disease in accordance with widely accepted protocols that are applied to all patients, more or less universally, sometimes without regard to their individuality. It is impersonal in its adoption of objective and technological means for diagnosis and treatment of illness. It is primarily drug- and surgery-oriented and often treats the symptoms of the disease rather than the underlying cause.

The alternative branch employs more holistic and unconventional diagnostic procedures and tradition-based nutritional, homeopathic, and herbal treatments, as well as physical manipulation and other techniques. The alternative branch tends to be more "patient centered" and is thus attracting more adherents. However, if you are in a car accident it is better to go first to the hospital emergency room to see a conventionally trained emergency medical doctor, rather than go to the naturopath, chiropractor, or aromatherapist. Clearly each approach has its particular benefits and appropriate applicability.

Business or Healing?

Further division arises because the mainstream branch also tends to be more commercialized, owing to the introduction of corporate medicine, wherein the physician is actually paid by the patient's HMO (health maintenance organization) or PPO (preferred provider organization) insurance plan. Naturally, corporations desire profits and therefore encourage the limiting of medical treatment. (You know, the 60-second consult with the doctor.) Thence we are confronted with a very important and fundamental question: Is medicine a healing profession, or is it a business?

The truth is that it is a healing profession that has been converted into a business. This poses a real conflict for many doctors, and it has also induced many patients to seek alternations, both from alternative health care providers and also on their own, supported by the many self-help books, the Internet, and other sources. The resulting situation is far from ideal because many of the professionals that are the best trained to guide the health care system are now de facto employees of large profit-seeking corporations and are thus estranged from the very ideals that led them to their profession in the first place.

Consequently, many mainstream practitioners have become more interested in alternative medical approaches. Conversely, many alternative practitioners seek to apply scientific methodology not only in validating their traditional approaches, but also, when more holistic approaches fail, in providing relief for their patients. This trend is positive, and we are now seeing the synthesis of a new system called complementary or integrated medicine. However, both branches of health care, as well as the "new" branch of complementary medicine, need to respect the Hippocratic precept— knowing the relationship of the patient to his environment and diet if they hope to achieve their respective goals.

This book is about such a synthesis. It describes a revolutionary blood test that is consistent with the requirement set out in the ancient wisdom of Hippocrates and Lucretius and at the same time meets the efficacy standards of modern scientific technique. It answers the immediate and pressing health problems confronting both young and old in our population striving to meet the challenges of adapting to modern life. At the same time, it offers a practical solution for our society struggling to rein in the seemingly uncontrollable costs in caring for the health concerns of its citizens, now exacerbated by an increasing demand on the system posed by the growing numbers of baby boomers turning 50 and beyond, an age when health care costs accelerate.

This is a breakthrough diagnostic test, used for nearly 17 years in well over 100,000 cases worldwide. It has been empirically proven of profound health benefit to cases of uncontrolled weight gain, arthritis, migraine, chronic fatigue, intractable skin disorders, respiratory disorders, gastrointestinal disorders, and a host of other problems. The benefits may also embrace the increasingly common problems of infertility and hyperactivity in children and adults, which, like metabolic syndrome, have a common basis in disruption of the immune system. Thus it is truly a synthesis of the ancient wisdom of Hippocrates and modern scientific technique.

The message of this book is that you must eat in accordance with your own, unique, genetically based, biochemical makeup. If you heed this message, you will likely rid yourself and your family of most of the health problems common today.

In other words, this book shows it is possible to avoid fatigue, migraines, arthritis, weight problems, hyperactivity and attention deficit disorder, skin problems, breathing difficulties, weakening of the immune system, infertility, and others. It is possible to do so merely by accurately finding out what foods, food additives, chemicals, and even common drugs, are causing your problems, and then avoiding such "offending" substances accordingly.

The ALCAT Test

As mentioned, the way to obtain this information is through a simple blood test. It is called the ALCAT test. This test has been scientifically validated in the lab and in university and other clinical studies in several countries, over many years. It has been field-tested on well over a hundred thousand people, and most of them have been able to regain control over their health and their lives. The results are based on your own unique genetic and biochemical makeup. Thus it provides a treatment plan that is unique for each individual. It does not conflict with other diet plans or medical treatments. It has the potential to rescue society from the otherwise uncontrollable and devastating health care cost increases it now faces.

We describe, in simple language, how this process works and why it is of such great benefit. Many of the scientific studies are explained as well as the case studies that illustrate the application of the test results to the most commonly encountered health problems. You will see how the food you eat, the chemicals you are exposed to, and the way you live your life—whether or not you exercise, have excessive pollution exposure, and so on—influence how your genetic information expresses itself. These influences either promote genes that promote health and well-being or promote inflammatory processes and disease Thus our genetic makeup can be viewed as our health potential. How we eat and how we live our lives determines how that potential is expressed. Food and nutritional exposures are important factors in determining gene expression.

The benefit of knowing this has the potential to greatly extend your "health span." It can give you more energy, freedom from pain, normalization of weight, a better mental outlook, and innumerable other benefits. This book can also help you better comprehend other current health concepts and thereby bring them into a more usable context.

Universal Acceptance

Skeptics ask, "If this new test is so beneficial, then why isn't everyone already using it?" The answer is that members of the medical establishment have a lot invested in the status quo by way of professional commitment, financial capital, and intellectual involvement. This means that when things change, some people lose out. This is the main reason why new discoveries are accepted slowly, especially in the field of health care.

There are many examples of professional resistance to change. This theme is often repeated in scientific history.

The most classic example, which every medical student learns, is the tragedy of Dr. Ignaz Semmelweiss, an Austrian physician who, during the 19th century, proposed that doctors wash their hands before delivering a baby, especially if they had just conducted an autopsy. Performing autopsies was much more common in Semelweiss' time than it is today as the then "modern" physicians, as they liked to consider themselves, would make every effort to link the cause of death to an observable anatomical or physiological occurrence, or abnormality, which they hoped to identify through this means of hands-on investigation. Thus, it often happened that a physician might perform a routine autopsy and then moments later go off to delivery a baby, without washing his hands in between. As obvious as this may seem today, in his time the idea was revolutionary. His observation that this simple sanitary procedure saved many lives upset the Austrian medical establishment of the day. They criticized and then ostracized him so mercilessly that he eventually committed suicide.

In addition, medical doctors are not trained very extensively in nutrition in general, and usually not at all when it comes to food and environmental sensitivities. Thus they tend, as do others, to look for answers within their own sphere of knowledge.

A common example is the long time lapse before the health profession realized the true cause of scurvy. For hundreds of years scurvy plagued sailors during long sea voyages. Despite the observation of a British Royal Navy admiral, Sir Richard Hawkins, in 1593, that the condition cleared when his men set ashore in Brazil and began to consume oranges and lemons, containing vitamin C, the connection was not quickly made. That sensible, right-thinking professionals can ignore an obvious fact is not only astounding, but surprisingly common.

Nonetheless, 200 more years would pass before lemons (then called limes) would be standard fare among British sailors. Even the British Navy's chief medical doctor reported after a well-controlled study demonstrating the obvious benefit citrus consumption had on the disease, this treatment still took another 40 years to be adopted. Why? Because the "experts" of the day ascribed the cause of scurvy to a contagious miasma. Thus despite the evidence staring them in the face, the possibility of a dietary cause was not taken seriously. Such is the strength of scientific prejudice that even science is ignored in favor of a baseless explanation, if that explanation is held true by the many.

One other recent example worth noting is that of a very progressive and tenacious Australian physician, Dr. Barry Marshall. After long and arduous effort, Marshall, during the early 1980s persuaded the medical profession that gastric ulcer was caused by a bacterial infection (*Heliobacter pylori*) and not the hypersecretion of stomach acid associated with stress, thus overturning a decades-old notion. His theory was, at first, rejected. Then, to prove his theory, Dr. Marshall first verified through objective methods, that he was free of gastric ulcers. He then intentionally infected himself with the bacterium, which, according to his prediction, did induce the disease. In a current article, in *Clinical Medicine* (March/April 2002), entitled "Heliobacter pylori: 20 years on," Dr. Marshall explains, "H. pylori alters gastric physiology to cause acid hypersecretion and peptic ulcer. Secondly, it damages the acid secreting mucosa leading to atrophic gastritis and gastric cancer risk."

The same intellectual prejudice cast its pall over determining the cause of beriberi, another disease of dietary deficiency, in this case vitamin B_3. It too was ascribed to the work of some unknown infectious agent because that was the dominant paradigm of the day.

Usually it is of benefit that the scientific community demands rigorous proof before adopting a new concept. However, sometimes, as in the examples just cited, new concepts are rejected not because they lack proof to support them but merely because of professional prejudice; sometimes because the discoverer is not part of the "in" crowd, and other times because it just steps on too many toes. Such resistance to change, for whatever reason, can also cause significant suffering and loss of life.

One of the more embarrassing medical fiascoes caused thousands of lives to be sacrificed, extensive human suffering, and financial loss. It arose because of the deadly combination of corporate greed and scientific prejudice. Hidden and concealed from public reports is the professional blindness that allowed a misguided search for the cause of a strange neurological disorder, dubbed SMON, *subacute myelo-optico-neuropathy,* a disorder affecting the nervous system, causing progressive paralysis and possibly a slow painful death. It broke out in Japan in the late 1950s. Searching for its cause spurred the most expensive research effort ever associated with a single disease in all of Japanese history.

Many patients suffering from a neurological condition were prescribed a particular drug. By the time it was realized that the very drug used to treat the condition, was itself the very cause of a more serious form of the disease, it had taken 11,007 victims, several thousands of whom died. Ceiba Geigy (who has since merged with Sandoz and then changed the company name to Novartis, well-known today as the manufacturer of Ritalin) had received numerous reports of its drug's dangerous side effects from other markets, but concealed this fact from the frustrated Japanese investigating teams. That the drug was sold under two different brand names, Entero-vioform and Emaform, further obscured, and thus perpetuated, the problem.

The story of this tragedy is told in great detail by Professor Peter Duesberg, of University of California at Berkeley, in his well-researched book, *Inventing the AIDS Virus* (1995), and we refer readers there for more details.

Professor Duesberg writes, "For fifteen years the syndrome was mismanaged by the Japanese science establishment, where virtually all research efforts were controlled by virus hunters. Ignoring strong evidence to the contrary, researchers continued to assume the syndrome was contagious and searched for one virus after the another. Year after year the epidemic grew, despite public health measures to prevent the spread of an infectious agent. And in the end, medical doctors were forced to admit that their treatment had actually caused SMON in the first place."

Does this mean that medical doctors are inept, unable, or unfit to assist us in our health concerns? Of course not. Most doctors are well meaning and willingly sacrifice for their patients. It means only that doctors, like the rest of us, are only human. They are subject to the same prejudices, weaknesses, and shortcomings that may affect anyone.

Therefore, we all should also take responsible for maintaining our own health. This does not mean we should self-prescribe medications or ignore our doctor's advice, but we should live a healthy lifestyle and, as much as possible, prevent the occurrence of illness in the first place. It also means that sometimes it is also necessary to do our own research.

As Regina Herzlinger from the Harvard School of Business writes in her 1999 book *Market Driven Health Care,* "Doctor, wake up and smell the decaf lite cappuccino. Well-informed mastery-seeking Americans are no longer going to put doctors or anyone else up on a pedestal. Rather, the patient will make the doctor their partner in the health care process."

In this regard, you don't have to wait for every member of the scientific community to accept that foods and other substances, even generally healthy foods, can account for such a wide range of common illness, as well as premature aging, before you take advantage of this breakthrough test. You can benefit from it today, as have many of the world's best athletes, well-known celebrities, and thousands of others who are concerned with optimizing their health, performance, and well-being.

No doubt you will see yourself or family members in many of the remarkable stories that follow. We hope this will lead to greater control of your life and will improve the life of your loved ones.

At this point we would like to introduce a letter from the golf pro at the well-known Pebble Beach Country Club in California, who exemplifies the advantages of knowing which foods are safe and which he needs to avoid. His experience with this test is typical of many patients and illustrates several points that will later be raised in this book.

January 14, 1999

Dear Roger,

My exposure to what the ALCAT test is and the positive experience it can bring to one's life is exciting to address. I remember first reading about athletes gaining performance benefits after following "their" rotation diet. This certainly got my attention because as a professional golfer, I noticed how eating within a tournament round had dramatic consequences. Almost without exception, fatigue and clouded thinking would result following food consumption.

It was three years ago in some health magazine article when I first read of the test. AMTL Corporation sent me a "for physician" booklet that I took to my doctor right away. He dismissed the valuable material without even looking at it and said, "You are healthy and don't have food allergies." Unfortunately, I went with his opinion and did not follow through some other means to get the test done. Thirty-six months passed when a fellow golf pro asked me, on the putting green before a tournament, if I had heard of the "ALCAT test." This was an angel's message. The next day I had AMTL send me the testing package and book, then ordered my doctor to send my blood sample to Florida. That was a second and final opinion, which was a godsend.

Once the book *Your Hidden Food Allergies Could Be Making You Fat* arrived, things changed. It opened my eyes to how all these symptoms I had been experiencing could be related to "my" own food sensitivity. Everything made sense. The explanation of impact starting in childhood and continuing into adulthood was enlightening. All these exciting insights had to be shared first with my family —because of possible common genetic-code-inherited-at-birth reasons. I could not wait the 24 hours for the test results to return and get rolling on some results.

Now, some 77 days later and after faithfully adhering to the rotation-and-elimination procedure, everything in the book came to life. Even though the initial thrust was all about the increase in performance and health, which was clearly received, I also lost 21 lbs. of fat. The change in fat-to-muscle ratio was readily apparent in the mirror and [in]wearing clothes not worn in 11 years. My wife kept threatening to give all these brand-new pants to the Goodwill—"I'm back in my closet now!" I tell everybody, "I'm not a walking bee sting anymore" in a swollen fat suit. It's like a stuffed-up nose, which I had quite often, clearing up, now being able to use it for breathing again. These are results that bring back functions that are sound and basic—I got to have it!

As for this change in eating habits—for true nutrition being anything difficult to do— the choice is clear. Sure, planning ahead is now absolutely necessary, but being lazy and not paying attention can get you stuck in the mud in more ways than one. Traveling in a clean efficient sports car burning high-octane fuel or a muddy, gas-guzzling dump truck—take your pick. The way it turns out, it is not a matter of willpower or pushing away anymore. Your instrument— your body—responds immediately by not craving sweets and carbo starches (dead foods). Fast overeating, as my family knew me well for, naturally does not occur because satiation is happening. Can you imagine that!

Actually, this whole thing has been two tons of fun to watch in action. As I said, everything pointed out in the book turned out to be true in fact. Early on my wife and kids were quite skeptical because they had to listen to the battle I had over the extra weight and inches of fat for nearly two decades. I remember reading and laughing in the first pages of the book exclaiming, " See . . . It's my body chemistry that keeps making me a pig . . . I can't help myself"; "Now I understand what's gong on here." I could go on and on about this experience just like a golfer giving you that play-by-play of his entire round of golf. Well, *I* enjoyed it! There is an entire world of people suffering needlessly from not knowing this valuable information that AMTL Corporation can provide and let you live again. It's like the movie *It's a Wonderful Life*. The impact things can have in changing the course one goes through just by plain living and communicating. That is the reason for this letter—I would love to be an instrument of communication to others who could share my enthusiasm for better performance of living. I can't wait now to see the positive changes this education about basic nutrition will have for everyone else.

Many times my work involves the training of influential people and CEOs to Fortune 500 companies in a recreational setting. Just think, if they only knew what kind of performance and health benefits could be delivered to their subordinate workforces. Ultimately, bottom-line results would actualize in cheaper insurance costs, better care, and a higher overall alertness in their employees. . . .

Most Respectfully,

Patrick Holiman

In this introduction, we have touched on the *what* of food and chemical intolerance. In the next chapter we'll discuss more about the *why* of this widespread phenomenon.

CHAPTER 1

A Medical Breakthrough for the 21st Century

I've tried all kinds of diets and I never kept the weight off. Now I'm losing weight without being hungry. I don't know how this is working, but it's working.

—Diane, housewife, Florida

The insulin dosage for my diabetes dropped from 90 to 25 units within one week.

—Joan, high school teacher, California

My panic disorder cleared up completely.

—Rose, registered nurse, Florida

After receiving my ALCAT results, I have been headache free.

—Isabel Le Doux, Indianapolis

Every season, I used to be constantly sick and struggle with colds and flu. Now I'm totally healthy in spite of a big flu that got half our team.

—Christian Mayer, World Cup winner,
Austrian Ski Team, Salzburg

I lost about one-and-a-half pounds each week without changing my activity level or consciously reducing portions. I
found I wasn't as hungry and had fewer cravings.

—John Magauran, M.D., general practitioner,
Honolulu, Hawaii

How were these people able to achieve the optimum
health and ideal weight that eludes so many of us
today? What miracle pill or treatment transported
them from a life of excess weight, physical pain, or mental
distress to a life of maximum health and normal weight?
Many diets have become popular over the years, the most
recent being the high-protein diet. However, recent studies suggest that excessive protein intake significantly increases cancer risk. It also increases the acidity of the
blood, resulting in calcium loss and osteoporosis risk. Excessive dietary protein intake also damages the kidneys.
Once again, a balanced and sustainable diet, based on individual biochemistry, is the most sensible approach.
Proper diagnosis of food intolerance, a common but frequently ignored medical condition, made the difference
in the lives of these five people—and thousands of others
around the world.

In fact, proper diagnosis of food intolerance (also
called food allergy and food sensitivity) is helping cure a
wide range of health care problems from obesity to depression to diabetes. When you remove the specific foods
that disturb your body's unique biochemistry, you can heal
and operate at peak performance without nagging, even
sometimes life-threatening symptoms. According to medical experts, recognizing and treating food intolerance
may be just the medical breakthrough needed to treat the
growing number of health problems that plague modern

people. Here are a few of many comments made by doctors who have treated illness by showing their patients what foods are making them sick:

Food intolerance and allergy have become an increasingly serious problem in recent decades. Food allergy might be the cause or aggravation of almost any disorder, and, often enough, it is the cause.

—James C. Breneman, M.D., *Basics of Food Allergy*

It's a great disappointment that doctors don't bother to consider food intolerance, because removing certain foods from certain people's diets can be helpful with so many problems.

—John W. Gerrard, M.D., former professor of pediatrics, University of Saskatchewan, Canada

Failure to recognize and control food allergy throughout life accounts for much unnecessary morbidity, invalidism, and even mortality.

—Albert H. Rowe, M.D., *Food Allergy: Its Manifestation and Control*

A New View of Food

At 56, Joan was dying. Her diabetes was out of control, and she was 72 pounds overweight. No drug, diet, or therapy had any impact on her deteriorating health. One of her sisters had recently died from multiple sclerosis, and Joan's husband didn't want to lose his wife at such a young age. He insisted that she immediately go to the hospital for intensive medical attention. Joan said she trusted only one doctor with her life, so she flew across the country from San Francisco to Baltimore for an appointment with Dr. Barbara Solomon, a relative. On reviewing Joan's condition, Dr. Solomon suspected that food intolerance was contributing to her health problems. She explained that Joan's body was quite possibly reacting to defend itself against common, otherwise "healthy" foods. Dr. Solomon immediately ordered a simple blood test to find out whether this was the case and, if so, exactly which foods were aggravating Joan's diabetes and obesity.

Within two days Joan learned something that completely surprised her—foods she ate every day were killing her. In fact, her body's biochemistry was reacting adversely to nearly 50 out of 100 common foods, including olives, nuts, wheat, certain fruits, white sugar, meats from domesticated animals, and some types of fish. Although she did not understand how these usually wholesome foods could be making her sick, Joan nonetheless followed the doctor's orders and eliminated from her diet all her "allergenic" foods. She was stunned when her insulin requirement dropped from 90 units a day to 25 units within one week— an "extraordinary and life-saving change . . . nothing short of a miracle," according to Dr. Solomon.

What's more, within six months of removing her reactive foods from her diet, Joan, who stands 5 feet, 4 inches, lost 37 pounds—dropping from a dangerous 192 pounds to a comfortable 156. Her family had always eaten a healthy diet—including organic foods from the health food store, fresh herbs from the family garden, and fruit from their own trees. Nevertheless, once she stopped eating the foods to which she had intolerances, Joan felt better than she had in years. She says, "My mood swings have disappeared, I handle stress better, I have more self-esteem, and I have more energy in my personal life and teaching career. I have even become more faithful with exercise, whereas previously I would choose a good book on the couch over a walk to the park. I can't say enough good things about the food intolerance test. I don't even want to think about where I'd be today without it."

The Key to Maximum Health
and Minimum Weight

The diagnosis that literally saved Joan's life—food intolerance—has already helped improve the health of hundreds of thousands of other people around the world who suffer from a wide range of symptoms and illnesses, including diabetes, arthritis, obesity, chronic fatigue, migraines, panic attacks, intestinal problems, and childhood illnesses such as ear infections, attention deficit disorder (ADD), and bedwetting. Food intolerance is not a medical diagnosis you hear every day—yet it's more common than most of us (including many medical professionals) realize.

Although a complex biological process, food intolerance is, simply stated, an individualized biochemical sensitivity to foods that are otherwise wholesome and harmless. This sensitivity causes the immune system to react as if it were protecting the body from an enemy such as a bacteria, virus, or parasite. This reaction to common foods causes intricate systems within the body to begin malfunctioning. One abnormal function triggers and impacts the next, like a series of dominos falling, until the slow dance of dysfunction surfaces in one form of ill health or another.

This series of malfunctions begins when a person eats the foods that he or she cannot tolerate. Usually protein molecules or one or more chemicals (either naturally occurring or synthesized by humans) in these particular foods cause a complex series of reactions, which eventually cause the white blood cells to react and sometimes "explode." When they explode, they release packets of chemicals that go to work to defend the body against the "invader."

If these powerful chemicals have too many enemies to fight (the result of regularly eating your reactive foods), they can leave a trail of destruction. Several adverse reactions can result, such as leaky blood vessels, increased production of mucus, chronic inflammation of tissue, contraction of smooth muscle in the lungs, intestines, and stomach, and general disruption of biochemical processes.

These side effects can wreak havoc in the body, eventually impacting almost any organ and bringing about disease symptoms. Like our fingerprints, our food sensitivities are not the same as those of any other person (except by chance). Whereas one person can eat all the chicken he wants without adverse effects, another might break out in hives the next day, develop a migraine two days later, or land in the hospital if she eats so much as a drumstick.

Your Own Personal Poison

Many people confuse food intolerance with food allergy. Although the difference between the two is complicated, a simple distinction is that the person allergic to foods, such as peanuts, strawberries, or shrimp, reacts immediately—often with a rash or, in extreme cases, anaphylactic shock (a severe and sometimes fatal allergic response). This type of reaction to food is rare—less than 5 percent of the U.S. population exhibits what is called "true" food allergy. Food intolerance, in contrast, is often called the "hidden" food allergy, because you usually have no apparent immediate reaction when you eat a food to which your body is sensitive. In fact, the body's reaction to offending foods usually occurs in small steps. Each step leads to the next until at some point, the body reaches a breaking point—the final straw.

At that point, the body reacts by developing one or more of a wide range of symptoms and diseases such as obesity, arthritis, diabetes, gastrointestinal problems, sinus conditions, or migraines. The cellular changes may be so subtle and discrete that you don't associate them with a food you eat regularly; yet if you continue to eat this food, your physical health will progressively deteriorate. Doctors who understand the profound relationship between food and health, and who understand and respect the destructive forces of food intolerance, can offer relief. No drug, no medical therapy, and no diet alone can improve your health or help you lose weight if you continue to bombard your body with your own personal poison.

No drug, no medical therapy, and no diet alone can improve your health or help you lose weight if you continue to bombard your body with your own personal poison.

Joan and other sufferers who struggle for maximum health and normal weight (and sometimes for their lives) have learned that food intolerance is indeed their health problem—or an important part of their problem. Unlike the rarely occurring "true" food allergy, where symptom onset is immediate, food *intolerance,* often called "hidden" food allergy, or food sensitivity, is common. Current research from a variety of sources estimates that between 30 and 90 percent of the general population suffers from food intolerance, which may manifest as relatively mild acne or a stuffy nose to conditions as deadly as diabetes or asthma. Growing evidence demonstrates that food intolerance may also play a significant role in the greatest health epidemic faced by the medical community today—obesity. As the correlation between biochemistry and overweight becomes increasingly apparent, it's not surprising that intolerance to foods contributes to the biological glitch that makes so many of us too fat for our own good health and self-esteem. Your body's reaction to your allergic foods is predictable and consistent. To prevent the predictable consequences of eating allergic or reactive foods, one may simply eliminate them from the diet.

Like Joan, most people find it hard to believe that otherwise healthful foods could contribute to health problems. After all, most of us were raised to believe that good foods build strong bones, enrich blood, and keep the doctor away. It seems illogical that a glass of fresh milk, iron-rich beef, or an innocent apple could have the potential to make us sick. Yet when Walter drinks milk, he develops severe gastrointestinal problems; when Barbara eats a hamburger, she gets a migraine; and when Sue eats even a little bit of apple, her eczema returns. Often people don't believe the reality of food intolerance until they see the impact in their own lives.

Arthritis Sufferer Finds a Simple Cure

Carla first heard about food intolerance in the office of Dr. Jay Sandweiss, an internist in Detroit. Sandweiss was on the long list of doctors she'd seen in her desperate search to find relief from worsening arthritis. During Carla's first office visit, Dr. Sandweiss recommended the ALCAT test for food and chemical intolerance. When the test results showed that Carla was intolerant to chocolate and green beans, she thought she had wasted her money again. She left the office feeling let down by yet another medical practitioner.

Dr. Sandweiss didn't hear from Carla again until a year later when she wrote to explain that she'd thought he was a quack when he recommended the food intolerance test. Then, when he told her she was allergic to common foods and that they were contributing to her worsening arthritis, she was sure he was giving her a bunch of baloney. But one day she thought,

> Well, I've spent the money, I might as well try eliminating these foods and see what happens. And to my amazement my arthritis went away. I had no pain, and I was able to do needlepoint and all the things I hadn't done in years. Then I got overconfident and ate some chocolate at Christmas. When I woke up the next day I was crippled in pain again. Now I keep my diet cleaned of all my reactive foods and I'm totally cured. You changed my life and I can't believe the food I was eating is what was causing my health problem.

Food Intolerance Saves the Day . . . and a Life

No one has to tell Sharon how insidious food intolerance can be at destroying health. After eating a bit of salad one day, the chronic stomach pains she'd had for years—cramps, bloating, and gas—escalated to the point of panic. Her stomach hurt so badly she thought she was going to die of a diseased colon—as her father had six months prior. "My health was deteriorating so rapidly that I was sure I was next," she remembers. A gastrointestinal specialist performed a test and found that her entire colon was inflamed and covered in ulcers and polyps. He put her on medication, which turned her skin yellow and made her feel worse.

As luck would have it, a dietitian she was seeing at the time to help her lose weight recommended she be tested for food intolerance. The test showed that Sharon had many food sensitivities—so many in fact, that she was left with only a few foods to eat, including turkey, lamb, tuna, squash, and spinach. Desperate to try anything that might make the excruciating pain go away, she embarked on her specially designed diet, which eliminated all her intolerant foods.

On the tenth day she felt like a new person. "I'll remember that day as long as I live—it was a euphoric feeling," says Sharon. "I immediately called my doctor to tell him that I felt better and was going off the pills. He scheduled a checkup right away. He was shocked to find my colon as healthy as any he'd ever seen. All the inflammation, ulcers, and polyps were gone. The food intolerance test saved my life. I would recommend this test for anyone and everyone."

Food Intolerance and Infertility

More couples are having problems with infertility. The number of fertility procedures increased by 27 percent between 1996 and 1998 in the United States, according to government researchers from the Centers for Disease Control and Prevention, reporting in a press release in February 2002. There are a number of explanations for this, and most of them involve chronic activation of the immune system caused by exposure to environmental factors, foods, and food additives.

When the immune system is activated, a particular cytokine released from macrophages (a type of white blood cells), interleukin 1, suppresses the production of luteinizing hormone and follicle-stimulating hormone, thus inhibiting pregnancy. Most likely, the body reacts as if it were suffering from a chronic infection, indistinguishable from a chronic food and/or chemical intolerance, and determines it is not a good time to become pregnant.

Dr. Lene Høj, an allergy specialist from Copenhagen, has seen about 50 female patients become pregnant after specific food elimination based on food sensitivity testing using the ALCAT test. Some of the patients had been infertile for as long as eight years. Remarkably, in most cases, pregnancy followed in just two or three months following dietary changes.

Dr. Høj believes that the inflammation caused by the immune system response to the food intolerance caused a swelling in the mucosal lining of the fallopian tubes, preventing the ovum's movement to the uterus. She has also tested males and observed an improvement in sperm counts, motility, and morphology following specific food elimination. She is hopeful about the benefits of food intolerance testing for treating infertility and intends to perform a prospective study to confirm her observations.

Food Intolerance and Frequent Infections

Doctors had observed for many years that patients with food intolerance were more susceptible to colds, flu, and other infections. A recent study performed at the University of Rome by Dr. Christina Mele and co-workers found that after the immune system cells in the blood were exposed to food substances that registered a reaction on the ALCAT test, they were no longer able to react to a stimulus that shows their ability to fight bacteria and other pathogens.

Zymosan, a product derived from a species of yeast, is used by laboratory scientists to determine the competency of white blood cells. If the white blood cells that fight infection are functioning properly, a zymosan "challenge," that is, exposing the zymosan to the white blood cells in the test tube, should cause them to release mediators, which are chemicals that induce an attack against the perceived pathogen. The released mediator combine with a chemical (luminol) that emits light, measurable by a sensitive instrument. The method of measurement is known by laboratory scientists as "chemoluminescence." Using this technique,

Fig. 1.1. Dr. Mele showed that immune system cells that react to a food (test positive on the ALCAT test) become less capable of protecting the body from infection.

Dr. Mele found that the stronger the ALCAT test reaction to a food, the less capable those white cells were of responding to a zymosan challenge later on (see figures 1.1, 1.2, and 1.3). The inference is that the immune system resources are being used to react against a food or chemical and are then not available to fight infections. When people discover which foods they are sensitive to, their immune resources are conserved and they then get fewer colds and flus.

Food Intolerance and Heart Disease

In the November 2001 issue of the *Journal of the American Medical Association (JAMA)*, Dr. Stanley Hazan reported on a study of 333 heart patients. He made the remarkable discovery that blood levels of inflammatory chemicals released by white blood cells were a far better predictor of heart attack than were cholesterol levels. In fact, he found that patients with the highest levels of a chemical called

Fig. 1.2. Immune cell competence following in-vitro challenge with ALCAT positive foods.

Fig. 1.3. Dr. Mele's study showed that the stronger the ALCAT test reaction, the "weaker" the immune system became.

myeloperoxidase (MPO), released by white blood cells, had 20 times greater risk of heart disease than did subjects with the lowest levels. "What is exciting is that this marker appears to be significantly better at predicting risk for atherosclerosis, or hardening of the arteries, than blood tests now used," noted Dr. Hazan. He cited that about 50 percent of heart attack patients have normal cholesterol.

Another study in the same *JAMA* issue, involving more than 3,000 subjects in Scandinavia, reported by Dr. Eva Lindmark and colleagues from Uppsala University Hospital in Sweden, that subjects with higher levels of interleukin 6 (IL6) had a significantly greater risk of developing heart disease. IL6 is also an inflammatory mediator produced by white blood cells, but it is also produced by adipocytes, that is, fat cells. The evidence is quite compelling that immune system activation is a major, probably *the* major, cause of cardiovascular disease.

Free from a Prison of Fat

The problem of obesity is so great in our nation that major health care organizations are scrambling to find an effective and healthy way to deal with what's been called "the fattening of America." Much current research on weight loss points solidly in the direction of a correlation between obesity and a biochemical glitch in the brain—a similar biological glitch to that created by food intolerance. Research already shows that people not only lose weight on a diet that eliminates their intolerant foods, but they lose fat, not lean muscle.

Although research clearly shows that eliminating badly tolerated foods from the diet is an effective weight loss approach, the greatest proof lies in personal stories of triumph over conditions that were ruining lives by trapping people in prisons of fat. Dianna's story has been repeated by thousands of weight watchers around the world. For years, Dianna had struggled with her weight, losing and gaining the same 30 pounds many times. She'd tried every popular diet and none were helping her lose and keep off weight.

Eventually she found herself 60 pounds overweight and feeling out of control. Fortunately, she met up with an old friend who had also struggled with weight. "She had lost so much weight that she looked like she'd lost another person," says Dianna. "I barely recognized her. I asked her how she lost her weight and she told me about food intolerance. She had eliminated foods that her body didn't tolerate and ate all she wanted of everything else, and she lost weight for the first time in years. It sounded too good to be true."

Despite her disbelief, Dianna scheduled an appointment to have her blood tested for her food intolerances, and was surprised to learn that she was sensitive to many foods, including the very foods she was eating on her many weight loss diets. Her new food intolerance diet basically consisted of all she wanted of beef, chicken, fish, eggs, spinach, cabbage, beets, carrots, celery, lettuce, walnut oil, and some grains. Within seven months she'd lost all her excess weight. "I lost the weight slowly, and I wasn't hungry at all. I was completely satisfied with whatever I ate. I don't know why this diet worked when everything else failed. I'm afraid to even question it, but it worked."

Rose was another lucky overweight person who learned about food intolerance and finally conquered her battle with the bulge. She was 160 pounds overweight and had tried every diet on the market. Then she learned about food intolerance, from a dietitian who had already helped many people lose weight. Rose had her blood tested and stopped eating the foods to which she was reactive, but ate as much as she wanted of every other food. She lost 100 pounds in six months and felt better than she had in years. "I have been on so many different diets over the years, but I felt different on this one. I felt very healthy and I had no food cravings. My energy level was intoxicating," Rose says. "I wished that I could bottle that energy and take a whiff every now and then."

World-Class Health

More energy and better performance is something every-one craves in our modern world with its endless list of "to do's" and daily stresses. But the idea of better perfor-mance takes on a whole new meaning when you are a world-class athlete competing in major sporting events, where a fraction of a second can mean the difference be-tween winning and losing. Just ask Christian Mayer, a skier with the Austrian Ski Team, who won the World Cup in the Giant Slalom event two years in a row and a bronze medal at the Winter Olympics in Lillehammer, Norway.

When his chronic stuffy nose began to interfere with his performance, at the suggestion of his team's coach Mayer went to see Dr. Stephen Schimpf, an Austrian physi-cian. Dr. Schimpf immediately tested him for food intoler-ance and found several sensitivities, including those to milk, wheat, tomatoes, and beer. After eliminating those foods, not only did Christian's stuffy nose disappear, but also his headaches disappeared, he lost 10 pounds of off-season ex-cess weight, and he had greater energy. "After the diet I was much quicker in the slalom and felt much stronger overall; and best of all, I'm still winning," he says. "At the end of every season, I used to gain 10 pounds. Now, with the frame-work of my food intolerance food plan, I can eat what I want and I don't gain even one pound. Also, I used to be constantly sick and struggle with colds and flu. Now, I'm to-tally healthy in spite of a big flu that got half our team."

Dr. Schimpf has since tested other members of the Austrian ski team for their food intolerances as well as many other Austrian sportspeople. "They have all had ex-tremely good results—they feel more energetic, keep off extra weight more easily, and perform better. In fact, many have gone public to explain the benefit they've received from the food intolerance testing. These Austrian athletes are absolutely convinced that knowing and avoiding their food intolerances is the way to improve their health and maximize their performance."

No Longer Sick and Tired

More energy and better performance is needed not just in the realm of world-class athletes. All of us need more energy to keep up with the demands of our modern world. Yet more of us than ever suffer from chronic, low-grade symptoms that sap our energy and make even simple chores pile up like so much deadwood after a storm. From our mid-afternoon slumps to chronic fatigue syndrome, too many of us are tired these days for this condition to be a coincidence. Something is clearly wrong. But what?

Many practitioners point their fingers at food intolerance. Why? Because when patients like Rose and Christian eliminate their intolerant foods they have more energy than they've had in years. After two bouts with the flu, Cleason (another example), could not seem to regain his strength. He became so tired that he missed days of work, then finally stopped going to work altogether. Luckily, his wife had learned about food intolerance when seeking a cure for her children's health problems. Cleason had tried many therapies suggested by several doctors, but not until he removed the foods he couldn't tolerate did he lose the excessive tiredness, regain his energy, and become able to return to work.

Spared a Lifetime of Illness

The diagnosis of food intolerance has helped not only adults; children also benefit from learning which foods and other substances, such as dyes and preservatives, cause adverse reactions in their bodies. A long list of children's health problems, including ear infections, attention deficit disorder (ADD), attention deficit hyperactivity disorder (ADHD), autism, headaches, and eczema can be linked to food intolerance. Dozens of research studies show how removing badly tolerated foods (and food chemicals) can improve children's health and even cure debilitating conditions.

Dr. Walter Ward, an ear, nose, and throat/allergy specialist in North Carolina, says that one of the most dramatic medical cases he's ever encountered involved a boy of 5, whose mother had brought him in for sinus problems. The child also had severe renal problems, which physicians at a highly respected hospital were trying in vain to treat. "Those medical professionals were following traditional renal therapy, but it was having no impact," says Dr. Ward. "The kidneys were just going, and the doctors were essentially watching the kid die." He consulted a colleague from the University of Miami, who recommended the ALCAT test. The child went off his reactive foods, and his health immediately took an upward turn. Within a short time his kidneys were functioning normally.

Breakthrough Medical Treatment

These are only a few of thousands of stories about people who turned their health around, even saved their lives, by knowing and eliminating their food intolerances. If food intolerance testing can help the Joannas, Carlas, Roses, Christians, and Cleasons of the world improve their health, then food intolerance testing may very likely be the breakthrough medical treatment of the 21st century. Especially when you consider the billions of dollars already spent on research, medical technology developments, increasingly complex surgical treatments, and pharmaceutical creations, it's shocking that we are sicker and fatter than ever. In the United States alone, 12 million suffer from diabetes, and 16 million from arthritis; more than 50 percent of the country's adults are overweight.

And that's just the tip of the iceberg. The health of increasing numbers of people worldwide is being compromised by medical treatments that aren't working. All the while, the answer to maximum health and healthy weight may be as near as your kitchen table. Stop eating the foods that overload your system and cause your body to attack the foreigners, and you'll enjoy optimum health.

Food intolerance testing and treatment is a simple, painless, nonsurgical, nonpharmaceutical approach to improving health.

It's almost too simple to believe. Further good news is this: Unlike "trying" prescription drugs, surgeries, or other therapies, and dealing with the often severe side effects, eliminating your reactive foods and seeing what happens poses no risk to your health whatsoever. Like Rose and Dianna, you may lose your excess weight and gain energy. Like Cleason and Carla, you may recover from illnesses that crippled your ability to live life to the fullest. Or like Joan and Sharon, you may find the cure to the chronic illness that not only forces you to live life in poor health, but is leading you to premature death.

Food intolerance testing and treatment is a simple, painless, nonsurgical, nonpharmaceutical approach to improving health. By properly diagnosing our food sensitivities, the impact on the health, health care costs, mortality, and quality of life of our nation's citizens could be truly profound. It could be just what an ailing society needs to live productive, happy, and healthy lives in what's sure to be an exciting and challenging 21st century.

Diagnosis: Food Intolerance

According to current researchers in this area, anywhere from 30 to 90 percent of the population of the United States is intolerant of one or more foods. This number is believed to be rising because of several lifestyle factors in the modern world. The health implications of food intolerance vary widely. Although your symptoms may be as relatively minor as a runny nose, your neighbor may have crippling arthritis, and your relative may be chronically overweight. Whether you live a life of minor, but chronic, health problems that only inconvenience your lifestyle, or you suffer from a health problem that is developing into a life-threatening disease, or if you're somewhere between these extremes, you should find out whether food intolerance is the culprit.

A new technology (the ALCAT test) can identify the exact foods that may be causing a person to be sick and/or overweight. This patented technology is a simple computerized blood test, which measures any changes to white blood cells in the presence of common foods. If the white blood cells become enlarged, burst, or shrink, these changes set the stage for serious health problems that develop immediately or perhaps years later.

If you're living a life of glowing health, unencumbered by any health problems, you may be among the lucky few who do not have an aberrant biochemical reaction to any food or food chemical. But it's time to find out whether common foods are causing or exacerbating your health woes and to avoid those foods if one or more of the following symptoms have become a permanent fixture in your life:

Acne

Anxiety

Arthritis

Asthma

Attention deficit hyper-
  activity disorder
  (ADHD)

Autism

Bedwetting

Chronic diarrhea

Chronic fatigue

Depression

Diabetes

Ear or other frequent
  infections

Eczema

Fatigue

Hay fever symptoms
  (year-round)

Headaches (tension type
  and migraine)

Infertility

Inflammatory bowel
  disease

Migraine

Muscle aches

Obesity

Panic attacks

Stuffy nose

Urticaria

Although these are some of the most common food intolerance symptoms, food intolerance has been implicated in nearly any symptom imaginable. Like many medical conditions, which may present themselves in a wide range of severities and intensities, food intolerance manifests in a wide range of degrees. What's more, it fluctuates. Sometimes a food-intolerant person will have a good day and be symptom-free, and other days he or she will be totally incapacitated by ill health.

This fluctuation can be explained by the existence, or lack thereof, of various co-factors, such as airborne allergens, which may cross-react with a food constituent. Hence, food sensitivities may also change according to seasonal patterns. For example, apples will cross-react with birch tree pollen because there is a chemical similarity with their antigens. Ragweed pollen may cross-react with cantaloupe.

Sometimes exercise may induce symptoms which would not otherwise occur, as in exercise-induced asthma. This is because the white blood cell membrane may be stable at normal body temperature but become unstable and allow inflammatory mediator release when the body temperature rises, even just by one degree centigrade. Reactivity will also by influenced by how large the "total load" of chemically related substances is. As will be seen later on, a major cause of food and chemical intolerance is the liver's inability to detoxify a chemical in a food, naturally occurring, or added to it. Thus food and chemical intolerance is often dose related. Small doses are tolerated whereas excessive doses can trigger a reaction. How well the detoxification enzyme systems in the liver are supported by nutrient-derived co-factors is another fluctuating and important factor. Thus, the quality and quantity of our nutritional intake will affect our sensitivities.

Whether or not the gut is inflamed, for whatever reason (spicy food, alcohol consumption, an active infection, or even a localized allergic response), is another important determinant of reactive to ingested food items. This is because a fully digested protein will most likely not trigger a reaction in the same way that undigested protein will.

We can see why this problem, being as complex as it is, has been so difficult to identify before the advent of the ALCAT test.

Evolution of a Valid Testing Method

Although people have long been known that reactions to foods can cause many unpleasant symptoms, the vast numbers of foods present in our diets complicate treatment. Once scientists recognized that food sensitivities are caused by multiple factors, the white blood cells seemed a logical place to look for change. Because the white blood cell population is a final common pathway of all the various pathogenic mechanisms, a test was needed to detect specific changes in these white blood cells that would identify a specific food as causing reactions.

As was stated earlier, food intolerance testing and treatment is a simple, painless, nonsurgical, nonpharmaceutical approach to improving health. In the 1930s Drs. Robert Cooke and Warren T. Vaughn developed a method for testing food sensitivities. They withdrew blood from the subject and, using the methods available at the time, counted the white blood cells. They then had the subject eat the food in question. Some time after ingestion of the food, blood was withdrawn for the second time and the white blood cells counted again. If the counts were appreciably lower, the food was considered reactive. The measurement resulting from Cooke and Vaughn's method was dubbed the leucocytopenic index.

Basing his work on Cooke and Vaughn's, in the mid-1950s an allergist in El Paso named Arthur Black studied changes in white blood cells challenged with an allergen and then viewed them under a microscope. He observed that some allergens caused the white cells to disintegrate and to release chemical mediators of inflammation. These allergens were confirmed to cause clinical symptoms in many cases. William and Mary Bryan, a husband-and-wife team from Washington University, later took up this work and the "cytoxic" test became quite popular for some time. However, this test was never really accepted by mainstream medicine because, it was argued, the results were subjective and not easily reproduced. Some feel the test was not given a fair evaluation because it posed a serious threat to the status quo in medical practice.

Around 1983, American Medical Testing Laboratories began research on an automated and objective method for measuring changes in white blood cells and other cells when the blood is exposed to a battery of test substances. Foods were the primary focus, although food colorings, food additives, environmental chemicals, certain drugs, molds, and other substances can be tested as well. The test, named the ALCAT test,* uses a specially designed hematology analyzer with results that are interpreted by a computer. This renders the test objective and reproducible, something that has been verified on several occasions.

Dr. W. M. L. Neetling, professor of biochemistry, and Dr. A. M. Kachhelhoffer, professor of medicine, at the University of Orange Free State in Bloemfontein, South Africa, conducted a research study in 1998 in order to test the reproducibility of ALCAT test results. They sent coded samples to a nearby lab that performed 1,300 individual tests, enough to obtain statistically significant data. According to the investigators' report, the result was that "the overall reproducibility of [the] ALCAT system adds up to 92.0678 percent, which makes the system acceptable as a screening model of testing allergy reactions in humans" (see the Bibliography of Selected ALCAT Test Studies on page 309). Physicians' offices can request reprints of numerous studies at no cost by contacting this address:

Cell Science Systems, Ltd., Corp.
1239 E. Newport Center Dr., Ste. 101
Deerfield Beach, FL 33487 USA
Tel.: (954) 426-2304
www.Alcat.com

---

*The name ALCAT was originally an acronym for the Antigen Leukocyte Cellular Antibody Test. The ALCAT test has changed dramatically and now measures a much broader range of reactions than the original test; however, the acronym was retained.

What You Should Know
About Food Intolerance

This book gives you the most comprehensive look at this astounding medical condition too long overlooked by medicine practitioners. To help you understand food intolerance and its possible impact on you and your children's health and weight, the following chapters will explore:

- The breakthrough study on the impact of food intolerance on weight and health
- The field of food intolerance, including what causes the problem
- How common foods can impact your body and make your health deteriorate
- Why you may not be aware of this condition
- The details of treating several modern health care problems such as obesity and chronic fatigue through food intolerance
- How a simple blood test can tell you within a few days exactly which foods and food chemicals your system cannot tolerate
- The stories of dozens of people whose lives are already brimming with good health because they learned about their food intolerances
- How you can get on the road to maximum health and healthy weight

You'll learn how to help your body adapt to the challenges of our modern world—and how a simple technology has finally been developed to deal with 21st-century health problems. Follow in the footsteps of thousands who have already learned that the foods they eat every day are keeping them from enjoying a life of optimal health. Discover and manage your food intolerances, and you too may finally experience the maximum health and normal weight you desire.

CHAPTER 2

Overweight: The Plague of Our Age

Without our ability to gain weight, humans as a species would never have survived. In the world of our prehistoric ancestors, the hunters and gatherers, food was not always plentiful. When berries and roots were in season and when wild animals were not hibernating, our ancestors ate well—and they fattened up. Then during seasons when food was harder to come by, they relied on their stored fat to see them through the lean times.

Two biological functions assisted them as they struggled to survive this perpetual cycle of feast and famine. When they had abundant food, their bodies efficiently stored fat, and when there was less to eat, their metabolism slowed to adjust to the smaller quantities of food. They were genetically programmed to adapt their metabolic rates to food intake. Those who survived were blessed with "fat-storing" genes, whereas those who lacked these genes perished. And the survivors passed their "thrifty" genes on to future generation—in other words, to us. These genes, which evolved slowly over thousands of generations, have not caught up to modern living and eating. We use the same genes to program our bodies to store concentrated sugars, processed carbohydrates, and adulterated fats.

Prehistoric Bodies in the
Modern Western World

Ironically, the same biological self-preservation mechanism that helped our ancestors store and retain fat—and thereby survive cycles of feast and famine—is one of the factors ruining our health, even killing some of us today. Thousands die each year from health problems related to obesity (an estimated 300,000 people die annually). Further, obesity is a contributing risk factor for four of the seven leading causes of death. Former U.S. Surgeon General C. Everett Koop stated that obesity is the second greatest preventable cause of death, right behind smoking. In his 1994 "Shape Up America" campaign report, Koop stated that excess weight is "one of the most pervasive health threats affecting Americans today." What's more, obesity is on the rise more than ever before in our history. According to Dr. Philip James, a leading Scottish authority on nutrition and chairman of an international task force on obesity, "Obesity is doubling every five years so we have an epidemic that is coming at the health service like a tidal wave."

Current statistics appear to confirm Dr. James's prediction. In 1996, a U.S. Department of Agriculture study revealed that at least 33 percent of all adults in the United States were overweight; that number increased to 61 percent in 1999 according to the Surgeon General. In late 2001 the Surgeon General's report said 27 percent of Americans are obese and 61 percent are overweight. And other calculations are even grimmer: According to a 1995 report by the Institute of Medicine, 59 percent of the adult population met the current definition of clinical obesity, which qualifies the disease for epidemic status.

We obviously weren't impressed by this encroaching epidemic, because we keep getting fatter. Just to compare apples to apples, consider the results of Harris polls from 1983 to current. Among people over the age of 25, 80 percent of Americans are overweight. This is up from 58 percent in 1983, 64 percent in 1990, and 71 percent in 1995.

Want to hear more? This year Roland Sturm, a researcher at the UCLA/Rand Managed Care Center for Psychiatric Disorders in Santa Monica, California, reported on the health care costs related to obesity. According to Sturm, obesity increases a person's health care costs by an astounding 36 percent and medication costs by 77 percent. The study also found that obese people have 30 percent to 50 percent more chronic medical problems than smokers or problem drinkers. Obesity increased the average yearly health care cost by $395 while smoking and heavy drinking resulted in $230 and $150 increases respectively. According to the U.S. Surgeon General in 1996, obesity cost us $117 billion—yes, that's billion with a "b"—annually. Now, it is considerably higher.

Now the bad news: Diabetes costs account for the majority of this amount. Those of you with relatives with diabetes understand how devastating this disease is. Type 2 diabetes is made worse by weight gain and is improved by weight loss.

At this point even we are weary of quoting statistics because ultimately real life has proven that Americans love to quote statistics but don't want to change their lives because of statistics. We want so badly to impress on you the seriousness of the situation that we find too many mind-numbing numbers. The numbers are all bad. This means it is time to stop trying to fix a system that has failed us and go back to basics. Each of us must find the foods he or she can safely eat and then eat them, not to "feel good" but to feel their best.

Adults aren't the only ones suffering from excess weight. A recently released Surgeon General's report says more children ages 12 to 20 are more overweight than ever before. According to the National Center for Health Statistics, one in every five U.S. children is considered overweight. No wonder the Institute of Medicine has declared war on the nation's "epidemic of obesity." Letting our kids choose their diets is like letting someone without a driver's license drive in a NASCAR race. Someone has to teach your kids how and why to eat, and their school isn't going to do it. In fact many schools have sold out to the soft drink and fast food companies, have candy sales to raise money, and door-to-door sugary sales to raise money for trips and projects. Asthma and diabetes are exploding in children's age groups. All this is happening because we taught them how to respond to name brand advertising rather than learn about their bodies needs and the dangers in the foods we eat. It is gut wrenching to realize that by age 5 most children have early signs of atherosclerosis.

In December 2001 the Surgeon General revealed that

> Overweight and obesity may not be infectious diseases, but they have reached epidemic proportions in the United States. . . . In 1999, an estimated 61 percent of U.S. adults were overweight or obese, and 13 percent of children and adolescents were overweight. Today there are nearly twice as many overweight children and almost three times as many overweight adolescents as there were in 1980. . . . Left unabated, overweight and obesity may soon cause as much preventable disease and death as cigarette smoking.

The Plague of Our Age

Why is the genetic self-preservation system we inherited from our prehistoric ancestors failing us in our modern world? One reason is that an important part of the feast and famine cycle is missing from the lifestyle of developed societies—the famines, which resulted in mandatory food fasts. No longer do we struggle through periods with very little food, thanks to modern farming techniques and food preservation, storage, shipping, and preparation methods. On the contrary, we live in a perpetual feast—eating seasonal foods all year long, consuming exotic foods grown around the world and shipped to our neighborhood grocery, and indulging in every conceivable convenience food that food manufacturers can dream up.

This means that our bodies are always on "store" mode. Rarely are they on use-up-the-excess-fuel mode—except, of course, when we go on low-fat diets in our perpetual, mostly hopeless, effort to lose excess weight. As most dieters now realize, this sets the body up to eventually cycle back around to nature's uncontrollable call to eat. The sad fact is that the body, as soon as possible after a "diet" (which the body interprets as a famine and therefore a threat), reacts by quickly regaining the lost weight—and then some—in preparation for the next food shortage, just as it did for our prehistoric ancestors.

An August 1996 article in *Scientific American* sums up our modern predicament well, stating that our growing problem of obesity can be blamed on "exceptionally thrifty genes—turned loose in an environment that offers easy access to high-energy food while requiring little hard labor." This brings us to another reason for America's excess of "saddlebags" and "spare tires." Whereas our ancestors had to work for their supper (from chasing down tigers to raising chickens), modern man can enjoy three meals a day plus snacks while exerting very little energy.

Dr. F. Xavier Pi-Sunyer, director of the Obesity Research Center at St. Luke's–Roosevelt Hospital in New York City, predicted in the same article, "we are going to see a continuing increase in obesity over the next 25 years" as standards of living continue to rise. Genetic heritage, too much food, and not enough exercise are among the many reasons why modern people in industrialized nations are facing the obesity plague. But one more reason is just now becoming clear to a growing number of health care practitioners—food intolerance contributes to the increasing problem of overweight, and the modern world "feast" is causing more people to develop food intolerances.

Fatter Than Ever . . .

There are many reasons why we are fatter than ever before. The modern Western diet consists largely of overprocessed, fatty foods manufactured by the ever-expanding food industry. These are known as "skeletonized" foods. With all or most of their nutrients removed by processing, they are little more than fat and carbohydrate skeletons of their original form.

Also, we live increasingly sedentary lifestyles, thanks in large part to modern technology. And the increasing prevalence of food intolerance is causing vast numbers of biological malfunctions that result in internal disturbances such as inappropriate fat storage, inefficient use of the stored fat, food cravings, and water retention.

A 1996 article in *Obesity Research* sums up the problem of obesity this way: "[The] modern Western lifestyle appears to provide the social and emotional conditions that favor maximum expression of underlying individual genetic differences in susceptibility to overweight." What this means is that our 20th-century Western lifestyle—with its highly processed foods, chemicals, pollution, stress, industrialization, and social structure—is triggering and exacerbating the body's instinct to prepare for and defend against famine. Today's lifestyle has wreaked havoc in the people who inherently have a genetic propensity to gain excess weight—which, statistically, includes most of us.

According to the Surgeon General's report, each individual body weight is the result of a combination of genetic, metabolic, behavioral, environmental, cultural, and socioeconomic influences. Interestingly, all these influences impact the development of food sensitivities. If food sensitivities are a common factor in all the identified factors associated with overweight, doesn't it make more sense to determine and eliminate the foods involved rather than try to take on the task of trying to change people's genes, their metabolism with drugs, their behavior with counseling, their environment, their cultural favorites, or the size of their paycheck? Maybe a better way to put it is that it would be cheaper and easier for us all if people would learn the foods they are able to eat regardless of the preceding factors. Let's take all these influences out of the picture by identifying the specific food demons.

Experts at a 1996 World Health Organization (WHO) conference said that the worldwide trend toward fatter people is caused in part by the increased use of machines, which lead to a more sedentary lifestyle. They added that the human brain biochemistry of modern people has not been able to adapt quickly enough to the reduced need for calories in our more sedentary lives, and that people are still eating as if they plowed farmland and milked cows for 10 hours every day. Studies cited by the WHO task force showed that with the many different populations around the world getting fatter, experts are dealing with a complicated environmental problem that needs an environmental solution. National survey data reveals that about 80–85 percent of American adults are overweight or obese—up from 43 percent in 1960.

People eat out often, they eat larger servings, and they seldom walk farther than the nearest car. Less than one third of adult Americans engage in the recommended 30 minutes of moderate physical exercise daily. Forty percent of adults in the United States do not participate in any leisure-time physical activity. Among adolescents, 43 percent watch more than two hours of television each day. We are so insecure about any exercise that we rush to gyms to hire personal trainers to teach us how to exercise. Long forgotten is the casual walk to the grocery or to church on Sunday. Instead of paying a personal trainer and then paying someone to mow your lawn, why don't you just mow the lawn? Walk to the grocery: You'll be surprised how much you save on your grocery bill if you have to carry the groceries home.

It's Just Not Healthy

Fat on the body is not, in and of itself, unhealthy. On the contrary, we all need some fat to keep us warm and provide a cushion for our bones and organs. Only when fat grows to excess do we have a problem. Excess fat is uncomfortable, unhealthy, and deemed by society as unattractive. Fat cells themselves release chemicals, like Interleukin 6 and TNF (tumor necrosis factor alpha) which are known to be inflammatory and thus cause cardiovascular and other degenerative diseases. Current research points out, obesity is unhealthier than we ever realized.

One study predicted that if obesity continues to increase at its current rate, every single man, woman, and child will be obese by the year 2030. Doctors who met at an international congress in Barcelona in 1996 said that obesity, with its often fatal complications, had become epidemic and could become a worldwide health disaster if not taken seriously and treated as a chronic disease. That prediction has come true much earlier than anticipated.

One theory on the dramatic rise of obesity is that overweight people do not fully comprehend the health hazards of being overweight and therefore are not truly motivated to find an approach that will help them take off and keep off weight. However, the health hazards of obesity are serious and are now becoming fully understood.

They include diabetes, heart disease, high blood pressure, high cholesterol levels, atherosclerosis, osteoarthritis, gall bladder disease, sleep apnea, and weakened joints. Research conducted by epidemiologists led by Dr. JoAnn E. Manson at Harvard University reported in a study of 115,000 nurses in 1995 that being even 20 pounds overweight invited disease and poor health. For every 2-pound weight gain, the risk of developing arthritis is increased by 9 to 13 percent. A weight gain of 11 to 18 pounds increases a person's risk of developing Type 2 diabetes to twice that of individuals who have not gained weight. Over 80 percent of the people with diabetes are overweight. Women gaining more than 20 pounds from age 18 to midlife more than double their risk of postmenopausal breast cancer. Obesity is associated with a higher incidence of asthma. Overweight and obesity are associated with increased rate of uterine, colon, gall bladder, prostate, kidney, and breast cancers. Obesity in pregnancy increases the risk of death to both the baby and the mother and is associated with neural tube defects, infertility, and low blood sugar.

In 1990 epidemiologists at Harvard conservatively estimated that treating the ailments that result from obesity in the United States alone cost $45.8 billion, and indirect costs due to missed work added in another $23 billion. In 2001 obesity and its ailments cost $117 billion per year. Experts of the WHO task force calculate that between 5 and 10 percent of the total health budgets of Western countries are involved with obesity, including treatment of the obesity-related illnesses such as arthritis, high blood pressure, back problems, and physiotherapy costs. These estimates are probably too low.

Beyond these serious health concerns, overweight people take a psychological beating from the social stigma of being overweight. Consider this commentary from a newspaper article written by a health writer from the *Boston Globe* regarding our nation's view of overweight people:

Americans have a curious relationship with fat. We're fat
and getting fatter. Our eating habits are unconscionable,
and our lifestyle is sedentary. We spend billions annually on
diets and exercise programs and then don't stick to them.
We turn to diet drugs. We resort to liposuction. We look to
magazines for advice and find articles that warn of eating
disorders alongside details of the latest semi-starvation diet,
or 'eating plan' in the current argot. We hate fat. We fear
fat. Fat people remind us of what we are, or what we could
become if we're not careful. So we distance ourselves by
making fun of them.

Is it any wonder that obese people are 20 percent less
likely to marry than their thinner counterparts? Research
also shows that the annual household income of obese
people is nearly $7,000 less than that of thinner people,
and they are 10 percent more likely to live a life of poverty.
All totaled, obesity and its ramifications have an obvious
depressing effect on self-esteem.

Despite the desperate search underway to find an effective way to battle the bulge, all the current research on
obesity is pointing to one fact: There is no magic bullet for
losing excess weight. Obesity is a complex problem, which
requires a change in our attitude about food and a change
in the way we eat. But in which way do we change our eating habits? "Eating differently" is precisely what distin-
guishes various diets. Some claim that cutting calories is
the ticket to melting the pounds away. Others claim low-fat
diets will help you fit into your favorite pair of jeans. Still
others point to high-protein diets as the path to slimness.
And that's only a few of the options for the person who
craves a life free from unsightly excess fat.

Yet the fact is that none of these approaches is working for the vast majority of the population. Although
people do tend to lose weight on the programs, they also
regain it over time. Recent clinical studies show that over
95 percent of people who use diets to control their weight

gain it all back within five years. Dr. Claude L'Enfant, director of the National Institute of Health's National Heart, Lung and Blood Institute, points out: "The difficulty lies in treating what is a very complex condition, affected by many social, cultural, behavioral, physiological, metabolic and genetic factors."

Fat and Unhappy

Although an estimated 80 percent of American adults are overweight, the percentage of people who are trying to lose weight is far greater. Their strategies range from over-the-counter diet pills to physician-supervised weight loss programs that integrate exercise and dieting with psychological counseling. Unfortunately, most people who need to lose weight are not succeeding. And there is not much scientific evidence to indicate that any of these strategies is consistently effective for most people. But still we try.

Among the many methods that dieters employ in their determination to be slim and healthy are low-calorie diets. At any one time, headlines can be found in several newsstand publications proclaiming new weight reduction diets and promising instant success: "Never Diet Again!" "Lose Weight Fast as You Walk!" "Blast Up to 49 Pounds Off in Only 29 Days!" The claims made by many so-called miracle weight loss programs are indeed tempting. But few have any research or long-term success stories to back them up. On the contrary, science is providing an increasingly convincing body of evidence to explain why it is extremely difficult for many people to achieve and maintain their desired body weight through low-calorie diets. The fact is that these "miracle diets" are as effective as the snake oil sold by 19th-century hucksters as a cure for everything from baldness to hemorrhoids.

We're here to tell you, "never diet again." Dieting is dumb, stressful, and counterproductive. It implies a temporary state, separate from "regular" eating. This hiatus from calories creates havoc in the body's feedback center. Forget dieting except that whenever you aren't eating what the body needs and can use, you are dieting as far as the body is concerned. Learn what your body needs and what you can eat . . . then eat it. Eating should be as impassive as filling your car with gasoline. The whole point should be to supply the energy for the trip of life, do not overfill the tank, and always be sure to put the proper fuel in the tank.

A Billion-Dollar Industry
on the Rise

Tempting claims like the ones just described are the reason the weight loss industry is a billion-dollar business—in fact, close to $30 billion in 1998. The 1998 sales of diet soft drinks is estimated at $12.5 billion, artificial sweeteners at $1.54 billion, health club memberships at $10 billion, commercial weight loss centers at $1 billion, low-calorie foods at more than $2 billion, and appetite suppressants at $1 billion. Add to this, books, tapes, seminars, doctor's office visits, and so forth, and the costs are staggering.

The weight loss industry is not making money because its methods *are* working. It's making billions of dollars because they're *not* working. The same overweight person will try the same weight loss program over and over, paying the often exorbitant rates for diet "secrets" until they finally give up and find a new diet program to spend their money on. This is the panic. Keeping dieters in the panic frenzy is very profitable for the weight loss industry as a whole. Just as restaurants profit when clients want a change of menu or are unhappy with service at another restaurant, weight loss clinics are content to recirculate the same 80 percent of Americans who are overweight.

People repeatedly go on these "low-calorie weight loss" diets with the blind faith that this time it will work; all they need is the willpower. They never stop to consider that the very premise of quick weight loss diets is flawed—and that the only thing guaranteed in the long run is their failure.

The weight loss industry is not making money because its methods are working. It's making billions of dollars because they're not working.

Statistically, when people lose weight on a low-calorie diet, they gain all the weight back within the first year. One reason that these diets are ineffective is because they are designed to have marketing sizzle, not practical guidance. After all, how many people would knock down the doors of weight loss clinics if their advertisements said, "Lose one pound a week by eating healthily and sensibly and by exercising daily"? Such ads simply wouldn't fly in America. We want stupendous results, and we want them now. So instead, the diet companies make claims such as "Eat all you want" and "Lose 10 pounds in 10 days." It is as though we are sure there is a miracle cure for obesity out there being suppressed by big business, and we jump toward every glitzy, scientific-sounding plan.

Folks, if there ever is a real breakthrough in controlling weight it won't be first marketed in the supermarket tabloids or on an infomercial. It will be tested, confirmed, and marketed through professionals who want to help you avoid complications and failure. Eventually your doctor will offer it as a practical aid to your weight loss plan. That is how the ALCAT test is marketed. The ALCAT test represents real science that radically differs from the conventional treatment of overweight that has made all Americans fatter. Our conventional treatment of overweight isn't working, but a lot of people are getting wealthy from it.

The weight loss industry is not making money because its methods are working. It's making billions of dollars because it's *not* working.

These ads recycle year after year, despite the fact that they don't work and despite the fact that they fly in the face of the reality of our body's actual biology. *Human Nutrition* gave this actual scientific description of how fat is gained or lost: Most medical experts agree that if energy intake and expenditure are not equally balanced, a deficit or excess of 3,500 kcal (kilocalories) normally causes a loss or gain of 1 pound of body fat. So, to result in weight loss, a person's food intake and activity level must cause energy expenditure to be 3,500 kcal greater than energy intake for every pound of weight loss

This description is something most dieters have heard before, right? Eliminate the magic 3,500 calories and a pound of fat will melt off. Well, listen to this additional, rarely discussed, explanation of weight loss from Gilbert Kaats, Ph.D., in the report of his group's study of the ALCAT test at Baylor Medical College, in the Spring 1996 issue of *The Bariatrician:*

> These figures assume that stored body fat is the source of the energy needed to make up for the deficit, which is the case in people who are overweight or obese. If muscle or other fat-free mass is being broken down to supply energy, however, then a deficit of only 580 kcal results in a loss of 1 pound of weight. This reflects the lower energy content of fat-free tissue, which is 70 percent water. Loss of fat-free tissue produces

the weight loss seen in starvation or severe malnutrition. Muscle loss is undesirable and in fact dangerous if there is appreciable loss, especially because it can affect the vital muscles of the heart.

Did you catch the significance of this explanation? It takes a deficit of 3,500 kcal to lose one pound of fat and only a mere 580 kcal to lose one pound of muscle, which is mostly water. So, if you've ever lost weight quickly on a low-calorie diet, what you've actually lost is muscle and water—not fat! This is no small fact. You may feel great when you look at the scale after a quick weight loss diet, but in the long run you will have done more damage than good. Even though you have lost weight, you now have a larger percentage of body fat. In other words, you are actually fatter than when you began the diet.

The question is, will the body attempt to conserve fat stores because it "perceives" the caloric restriction as a famine, and in so doing metabolize lean tissue? The answer really depends on other biological factors influences primarily by insulin activity. The likelihood is that if you're dieting to lose weight that the underlying biological factors which determine what type of tissue is metabolized (lean or fatty) will not be in your favor. The point to be made here is that the body under conditions of perceived starvation will utilize muscle so as to spare the metabolic energy required to maintain it. It is generally accepted that the weight lost in low calorie plans is up to 30 percent muscle mass.

Losing muscle tissue is a major health concern because muscle is the body-building tissue—the very tissue that burns calories most efficiently. Once you have shifted your percentage of lean to fat tissue, you'll find it even harder to lose weight because fat tissue requires fewer calories to sustain itself than muscle does. A reduction in muscle tissue is one reason dieters gain all the weight back and more as soon as they resume their previous eating habits. According to the *Harvard Heart Letter,* "typically as much as two-thirds of the lost weight is regained within one year, and almost all is regained within five years." This sets up a chronic dieter for the "yo-yo phenomenon."

Weight loss yo-yoing occurs when a large and rapid loss of weight is followed, as soon as the dieter relaxes control, by a gain in weight that is at least equally large and rapid. This occurs mainly because, in addition to a shift in lean-to-fat tissue, many people who achieve considerable weight loss experience, like their prehistoric ancestors, a reduction in their metabolic rates, and therefore a reduction in energy requirements, in their body's instinctual effort to defend against starvation. This allows the lost weight to be regained in a much shorter time than it was lost and means that the next time the person goes on a diet, losing the same amount of weight will take longer.

In addition to frustrating the dieter, recent studies indicate that "weight cycling" may actually be more dangerous than maintaining a steady but slightly increased weight over time. Yo-yoing has been shown to damage health in several ways, including increasing the chances of heart disease and heart attacks, gout, osteoarthritis, diabetes, certain cancers, and other disorders.

Problems with Popular Diets

Millions of people who desperately want to lose weight find hope through the ever-present variety of diets. A few favorites, including low-fat and high-protein diets, recycle on a regular basis. These weight loss notions fall into a whirlpool of increasingly contradictory information supplied by a number of reputable scientists.

One specialist will tout a low-fat diet as the key to weight loss; another will say that the answer is not eating less fat. As proof, the proponent may point to the fact that for the past several years many of us have been eating less fat, yet we're still fatter than ever. Some surveys show that the proportion of calories Americans get from fat has dropped about 8 percent to 34 percent of our diet since the 1980s. Yet the prevalence of obesity has risen during the same time frame.

A diet high in carbohydrates was the rage throughout the 1980s and into the early 1990s. This rage was fueled by athletes' eating patterns, such as the popular "carbo-loading" the day before an event such as a marathon run. But recently people have been forced to take a second look at the beloved high-carbohydrate diets. These highly touted carbohydrates turned out to be sugars and starches from processed foods that cause rapid rise in insulin levels with all its repercussions, as distinguished from healthy complex carbohydrates.

The terms *simple* and *complex carbohydrates* may be a little confusing. For metabolic purposes let's classify carbohydrates as to their glycemic index. This consistent evaluation of carbohydrates measures the insulin response to a food. The higher the glycemic index, the more insulin produced by the food. And the more insulin produced, the more fat is stored. Now current research indicates that high glycemic index foods have a similar effect as fat—excesses are just as likely to be stored as fat as is fat itself. In fact the elevated insulin levels will actually increase fat storage. Yes, insulin is a fat storing hormone. Plus, consuming high amounts of these foods will cause the body to produce more insulin, which causes blood sugar to drop, which not only stimulates appetite, but induces greater fat storage.

Compounding the problem of high-carbohydrate diets, especially simple carbohydrates, usually derived from processed foods and lacking in fiber is the fact that about 20 to 25 percent of the population is resistant to insulin. Insulin resistance impacts the body's ability to process carbohydrates properly, turning the sugars into fat and sending out an insistent demand for more carbohydrates. Insulin resistance may be the result of constant increased demand for more insulin production by the pancreas, resulting in the production of poor-quality insulin that is not capable of effectively transferring glucose into muscle cells; or, it may also result simply because the high fiber-lacking carbohydrate consumption increases blood sugar levels, and then insulin production, to such a high level that the tissue cells "down-regulate" the number of insulin receptors to compensate.

When the muscle and liver cells cannot receive the glucose, not only due to insulin resistance but also to storage capacity limitations occurring under even normal circumstances, the body stores it as fat rather than allow the blood sugar to remain dangerously elevated. High levels of blood sugar will bind with and degrade proteins in the blood producing substances called "AGES" advanced glycosylated end products. AGES, ironically, are associated with premature aging.

The high blood levels of insulin result in the rapid storage of fat, because the body interprets the elevated insulin levels as abundant glucose immediately available for energy. Interestingly, the same insulin that was ineffective at getting glucose into the muscle cell is seemingly quite efficient at driving fat into the fat cells.

High-protein diets, the rage in the mid-1970s, are back again in the 1990s. This time they pit themselves against the high-carbohydrate and low-fat diets. These high-protein proponents point out that protein is essential for replacing and maintaining muscle. The more muscle you have, the higher your metabolism and the more calories you'll burn, even when you're not exercising. Also, eating more protein can help you feel fuller longer, because protein takes longer to digest and be absorbed than carbohydrates do. As a result, dieters are less likely to nibble between meals or crave certain foods, which can reduce the overall number of calories you consume. However, too high an intake of protein may put undue strain on the kidneys. It can also cause acidification of the blood which will compensate by drawing minerals from the bones.

No matter how convincing the diet proponents are, the fact is that millions of people have tried these diets and are still fat. So no matter how rational the explanation of why a particular weight loss diet is the diet to follow, not one as yet has the success numbers to back up its claims. If anything, we should have learned by now that no one diet works for everyone. And until each person's individual biochemistry and food intolerance is taken into consideration, the battle to reduce America's bulk will continue raging.

Side Effects of Diet Drugs

So if low-calorie, low-fat, and high-protein diets don't work, then diet drugs must be the answer to our weighty woes, right? Again, we're looking for the magic bullet, the effortless weight loss approach that doesn't require us to become active participants in the acquisition and maintenance of our good health. So far the magic drug that lets us lose weight and continue our lives without lifestyle and dietary changes does not exist. Overweight is a sign that our lifestyles and food choices are inappropriate for our individual body chemistry. Overweight is beyond the scope of a "morning-after pill." Weight loss must become a personal crusade in which drugs serve only to temporarily distract us from hunger.

Many diet drugs used to treat obesity carry a heavy toll of side effects. For example, appetite suppressants help subside appetite but also stimulate the nervous system.

Many drugs of this class are chemically related to amphetamines and may cause similar side effects. When such side effects appear, they are hardly conducive to long-term use of the drug. But when the drug is discontinued, the appetite returns with a vengeance, again pointing out our need to discover the underlying cause rather than focus on the symptoms of overweight.

Over-the-counter diet drugs may contain phenylpropanolamine, which can cause nausea, headaches, nervousness, elevated blood sugar levels, insomnia, and rapid heartbeat. Because these drugs are obviously not innocuous, we must treat them with care. According to Steven B. Karch in *The Pathology of Drug Abuse*, second edition, patients have experienced chest pain, arrhythmia, arrhythmic sudden death, seizures, and psychotic episodes. Stroke has also been reported with some frequency.

Over-the-counter diet-aid manufacturers are notorious for throwing in a little of everything legal to convince you that all the bases are covered. Formulations may include ginseng, licorice, ephedra, caffeine, and chromium, to name a few. Such ingredients are used for their chemical or druglike effects and should be respected as such. Unfortunately, combining these concentrated drugs may compound the likelihood of serious side effects. For that reason, it's important that you know and understand all the drugs you introduce to your body and their potential risks. Another serious drawback of diet drugs is that although they may help you lose weight by suppressing your appetite, your weight loss is usually temporary because the root cause of the overeating problem remains.

There is no drug, nor will there ever be, a drug that selectively eliminates fat on the body without any effort on your part. At the very best maybe a drug may diminish cravings while you deal with eliminating unhealthy or allergic foods. Even then the elimination of fat is pretty much a matter of metabolism. You can choose to exercise and increase the rate of fat loss, or you can sit around bemoaning how much your doctor and his or her medicine cost. It bears repeating that any weight loss plan requires your cooperation and dedication to be successful.

Too many Americans hear the words "appetite suppressant" and think the words "weight loss." These are in no way synonymous. Appetite suppression is a chemical effect on brain hormones, weight loss is a modification of eating habits and exercise to result in calorie deficit. The only way that appetite suppressants and weight loss have any relationship is when one tries to restrict appetite while carefully excluding foods that are contributing to overweight.

Without this identification of foods and their restriction, long-term weight loss is a pipe dream. The most important point is that while losing weight by restricting excess calories, one must carefully supply nutrients to the body to build muscle, hormones, and enzymes. This usually results in my patients, after taking the ALCAT test, actually eating more food than they did previously. As they normalize hormone function and build muscle mass, weight loss predictably occurs. My observation is that one can lose weight using any healthy diet or program *if* one uses the ALCAT test to guide the foods eaten.

It is evident that no perfectly safe drugs are on the horizon for the control of appetite or weight. Each patient must evaluate the potential benefits and risks and make his or her choice. One thing is clear: Unless a drug is used to cure a disease, it is only a stopgap. Ultimately some effort must be made to determine the underlying cause of a patient's overweight and a curative treatment instituted to turn the risk-benefit ratio in favor of the patient. Patients whose excess weight is caused by food intolerance, need only use appetite suppressants temporarily to assist them in the speedy elimination of their culprit foods.

Why Can't I Get Help
from My Doctor?

Conventional medicine is locked into treating problems after they happen. The symptoms are evaluated and an appropriate medication prescribed to reverse or alleviate the symptoms. Few doctors can afford the time or expense of taking the time to teach. And ultimately what you need is to be taught what and how to eat.

Medications for appetite suppression have been used for decades mostly unsuccessfully for long-term weight management. There is often short-term weight loss, but as explained previously, medications do not alleviate the underlying problem. But as the demand for new medications to treat weight gain grew, the profitability of this new class of drugs tantalized the drug industry. New drugs were developed, and your doctor was encouraged to use these drugs approved for the treatment of overweight because the FDA approved them. Many doctors felt pressured to change their prescriptions to these "approved" drugs. Huge numbers of patients benefited from the drugs, and drug makers coffers swelled. Your doctor felt as though he or she had a reasonable option in helping you lose weight, one that the FDA had approved for weight loss. Even doctors who had previously shunned treatment of overweight began prescribing these drugs to help their patients.

Overnight this apparent gift of effective appetite control and weight loss turned into a health care catastrophe. Studies revealed dangerous effects on the heart from this medication that supposedly had been thoroughly studied before FDA approval of fenfluramine. Overnight the drug disappeared from the shelves of pharmacies. Almost as quickly the lawsuits began. Suddenly your doctor, who may have actually been treating you conservatively, found himself calling his malpractice insurance carrier in response to a subpoena for medical records by lawyers in a feeding frenzy.

To make a long story short, your doctor spent thousands of dollars, sleepless nights, and valuable time dealing with lawyers, courts, and depositions. Most of the doctors affected were eventually dropped from the lawsuits as the lawyers zeroed in on the drug maker. A multibillion dollar settlement was finally reached. But the point is that your doctor was punished severely economically and emotionally for treating patients with an approved drug. Is it any wonder why so many doctors don't want to put their professional, private, and economic lives on the line in the treatment of overweight?

As the picture of the treatment of overweight comes into focus, we have a population crying for help with weight management, complaining for lack of insurance coverage of weight management, who are willing to turn on the very people trying to help them. Subsequently, as malpractice insurance premiums soar each year it becomes more expensive to get well after you are sick. And to avoid exposure your doctor restricts his or her practice and resumes the safe practice of recommending that you need to lose weight and that you should see another doctor or dietician for help.

"Feel Good" Foods

Current thinking concerning food intolerance and obesity is that reactive foods trigger or inhibit the brain chemicals such as serotonin that control appetite and food cravings. When these potent chemicals are thrown out of balance in our bodies, we uncontrollably crave foods, especially starchy and sugary foods that will give us a quick surge of serotonin. These foods have a "serotonergic" impact on the brain chemicals; in other words, they trigger the same calming "feel good" effect as the serotonergic drugs. Because this is a short-term effect, within an hour or two we need another food "fix." In a sense, we are medicating ourselves with food.

Research shows that when foods to which we are intolerant are eliminated from our diet, the effect is similar to that of mood-altering drugs, only infinitely healthier— the brain chemistry returns to normal and the compulsive food cravings disappear. Researchers have not yet identified exactly why this occurs, but know that an important relationship exists between the allergic response of the white blood cells and platelets to brain chemistry. So it stands to reason that any disruption of the blood cells caused by allergenic foods could adversely impact the brain chemistry. With this safe, economical path to weight loss available to those with food intolerance, any rationale for the long-term use of drugs goes by the wayside.

Although hard evidence to prove this theory may be a few years away, medical practitioners do know that when patients remove foods they cannot tolerate from their diets, food cravings go away. They lose excess fat—and lose it naturally, without the expense and side effects of powerful weight loss drugs. Therefore, losing and keeping weight off begins by first identifying the individual's problem foods.

Modern Advances in Weight Loss

Currently, there is much hope and speculation in the medical world regarding genetic engineering. Using powerful new tools in molecular biology and genetic engineering, scientists in laboratories around the world are looking for cures for all kinds of disease, including obesity. Scientific theory regarding obesity says that we maintain our weight when our various metabolic feedback loops, tuned by whatever susceptibility genes we carry, settle into a happy equilibrium with our environment. The 21st-century effects of the economic, cultural, and lifestyle changes are propelling more of us—in particular, those with more genetic risk factors—into obesity. But genetic engineering researchers hope to someday find the hormone that will regulate metabolism and weight by, for example, signaling the brain that the body has stored enough fat.

Our understanding of how the body controls weight, or fails to do so, began to develop in the 1950s. It has gained momentum since late 1994, when the breakthrough was the cloning of a mouse gene that has a role in telling the body to plump up or slim down. The gene is called Ob, for *obese,* because obesity results when the gene does not work properly in mice. Abnormalities in the genes can result in an abnormal protein that interferes with the body's complicated and delicate balance of biochemical pathways controlling appetite and the processing of food.

The following year scientists identified the gene's protein associated with eating behavior and metabolic rate and called it leptin (after the Greek word for "thin"). Studies have shown that leptin apparently helps determine how much fat a mouse is carrying. If there's too much, leptin tempers the appetite and speeds up metabolism to burn more calories. Scientists gave mice daily injections of leptin and, in just two weeks, the mice lost 30 percent of their body weight.

However, by early 1996, before the dust surrounding this latest "breakthrough" had settled, the *New England Journal of Medicine* was reporting that, although it helped obese mice become thin, leptin didn't work the same way in humans. In fact, obese men and women appear to have plenty of leptin (four times more than people of normal weight), but they are unable to process its signal properly.

A follow-up study with human subjects showed that as food intake dropped, leptin levels dropped even further. The body's reaction to a decrease in food intake is to limit leptin's "stop eating" signal. This could be one reason why rapid weight loss programs don't work.

The early stage of genetic engineering has many drawbacks. The arena is so complex that scientists rarely find only one gene responsible for the problem in every person. Any single physiologic function is controlled by the interplay of several genes. For example, scientists have already located five genes that can cause rodents to gain weight. The best guess at this point is that obesity in humans is a polygenic disease, involving a number of genes that interact with each other and affect the biochemical pathways, which in turn influence our eating, metabolism, and physical activity.

And that is only the beginning of the problem. Once they discover the genes, scientists must then determine just how each exerts its power on our bodies. Then treatments have to be proven safe in animals, and finally in humans. Clinical trials must also show whether the gene is effective in people whose fatness is often due to reasons other than just genetics.

What's more, although to some degree genetics are clearly involved in obesity, they cannot be the whole story. Proof is apparent when we look at specific populations of people who have been taken out of their traditional environment. The Pima Indians, for example, are commonly cited by experts. Despite a common genetic background between the Pima Indians in Arizona and those who live in Mexico, American Pimas have a far higher incidence of obesity—in part because many eat high-fat foods, whereas Mexican Pimas subsist mainly on grains and vegetables. The American Pimas lead a more sedentary lifestyle, whereas their Mexican cousins still actively engage in growing their own food and livestock and exhibit normal weight patterns. In a study of fat-storing genes and their impact on society, conducted by Eric Ravussin, Ph.D., and Clifford Bogardus, M.D., obesity researchers working in Arizona for the National Institutes of Health, found more than 80 percent of the Arizona Indians weighed twice the national average. Most suffered from a host of medical conditions such as diabetes and gall bladder disease.

So the reengineering of a defective gene to make someone revert from fat to slender remains in the realm of theory and does not yet provide a practical solution. Considering all the challenges genetic researchers face, we can safely say that, despite encouraging advances, scientists are unlikely to discover miracle cures for the many chronic diseases that plague modern humans. Once again, effective treatment boils down to each individual—finding which foods we must avoid, making sensible lifestyle modifications, and starting a practical exercise program.

You Promise and You Promise

For decades now we have heard the promises of drugs and tests that will solve the problem of obesity. From genetic manipulation to "promising" new drugs, the hype strings us along as we nonchalantly gnaw on our poison. We are convinced that modern medicine will save us. It is easier to blame medicine's inability to solve the problem than to take charge ourselves. We have been coddled for so long that we feel inadequate to take care of our own bodies. Someone needs to stand up and say it out loud, "It's the food."

My experience tells me that we literally can eat to feel good or eat to feel bad. So why don't we all eat to feel good? The answer is that we don't know what to eat to feel good. We are content to eat what someone else makes taste good, without considering the ramifications. If you wake up in a good mood, you ate foods that supplied the needed nutrients to create the hormone balance to feel good. Likewise, if you wake up in a bad mood you ate foods and chemicals that limited or depleted the nutrient needed to make you feel good. I wish it were rocket science so you could be impressed at how smart I am, but it isn't. Your responsibility is to find the food balance that makes you the best person you can be.

The fact of the matter is that the odds are slim: There will never be a magic fat cure. We already know the cure, and we don't use it. It is kind of like the man who missed his train because he was waiting for a porter to load his bags for him. If you are going to wait for your doctor to offer you a cure, you are going to miss the train.

The Biochemical Connection to Obesity

Ever wonder why you have an uncontrollable craving for a particular food even though you may not be truly hungry? For decades, medical practitioners have blamed overeating and obesity on a lack of willpower, a lack of discipline, poor self-control, or psychological problems resulting from an addictive personality or traumatic childhood experiences. Obese people have been viewed as psychologically flawed, driven to overeat by neurotic self-defeating urges.

Those issues may indeed be part of the obesity problem in some people, but practitioners in the fields of psychology and medicine agree that such explanations are not valid for the more than one half of the adult population who are overweight. Virtually no scientific evidence supports these explanations or suggests that people who struggle with weight are any different psychologically from those who do not. Despite the absence of data, this stereotype persists among the public as well as within the medical community.

Many researchers in this area are convinced that obesity isn't a failure of will, but a chronic medical condition with complex biomedical roots. According to the Harvard

Medical School's *Harvard Heart Letter* (March 1994), "Medical researchers and weight loss experts no longer regard being overweight as a simple failure of willpower. Instead, obesity is increasingly considered a chronic disease, like hypertension or diabetes." The fact is that almost 50 million Americans are dieting right now and, statistically, 95 percent of them will fail—so logically, there has to be another reason why people are too fat and why they can't lose and keep off weight.

Recent advances in research have opened a new chapter in our understanding of obesity. Now new and promising research points to the effects of our powerful brain chemicals on our ability to lose and our propensity to gain weight. After almost 20 years of research on the relationship between brain chemistry and eating behaviors, Dr. Sara Leibowitz, a neuroscientist at Rockefeller University, found that disturbances in eating behavior reflect disturbances in brain chemistry. What we eat, when we eat, and how much we eat is determined by the type of brain chemistry we have, not the type of personality. These findings may at last lead to better ways to stop the powerful forces within our body from working against our best efforts to shed unwanted pounds of fat. The search is on for ways to correct these biochemical abnormalities.

To understand the complex biochemical forces that control our actions, we can benefit from knowing something about our brain chemistry. To start with, real hunger signals come from an area of the brain called the hypothalamus, which controls the balance between the body's need for food and its use of energy. The hypothalamus is the brain's nerve control center for many metabolic functions crucial to appetite control. It sends out powerful chemical messengers, called neurotransmitters and hormones, which influence when we eat, how much we eat, and what we eat.

The ideal way for us to approach our diet is to eat only when our appetite is stimulated by hunger and to stop eating when the appetite is inhibited at the appropriate point by the sensation of satiety. Recent research indicates that our ability to integrate our internal and external stimuli to achieve this depends on our chemical and physiological makeup. Normally chemicals in the brain signal whether we are hungry or full. A defect in the system could lead to overeating.

Your brain is the controller of food intake, receiving signals and sending signals, and adjusting the balance between metabolism and storage. We each have a number of specific neurotransmitters that are known to be involved in the integration and control of hunger and satiety, including gamma-aminobutyric acid (GABA), norepinephrine (noradrenaline), serotonin, dopamine, and histamine. Also, several neuropeptides (regulatory peptides able to affect the nervous system) are known to be involved, including neuropeptide Y, ß-endorphin, dynophine, growth hormone-releasing hormone, and galanin. All these stimulate food intake when injected into special regions of the hypothalamus. For example, if you skip a meal or eat a very low-calorie diet, galanin sends one very persistent message: Eat and store fat. When we eat certain carbohydrates, levels of serotonin increase and we feel better. When operating at optimum levels, the body naturally keeps serotonin levels high and block galanin overproduction.

Other important players in obesity include hormones. Brain-made hormones called endorphins, and certain amino acids (the building blocks of proteins) both act directly on the hypothalamus. Scientists have shown in animal experiments that high levels of brain endorphins affect the craving for fatty foods. Obese animals were found to have higher levels of endorphins in their hypothalamus and larger appetites. The hormone insulin controls blood sugar levels and signals the brain that the body has been fed. After a meal, insulin surges into the bloodstream, ordering our cells to suck up glucose and store it, and to absorb amino acids needed to build muscles and other tissues.

When insulin metabolism goes awry, as it can when you eat a food to which you are intolerant, levels of fats in the blood also go awry and you crave simple sugars. When you eat too much sugar and carbohydrates, the body releases insulin to bring down your blood sugar levels into the normal range. One way this occurs is by pushing sugar out of the bloodstream and depositing it as fat. This system served our prehistoric ancestors well because it helped ensure that they had the necessary fat reserves to make it through the next famine; however, this highly individualized insulin system is working against modern humans' ability to maintain an ideal body weight.

Thyroid: Mr. Metabolism

Hypothyroidism may be one of the most underdiagnosed conditions in America. It is estimated that millions of Americans are walking around exhausted, cold, losing their hair, feeling like they are going crazy because their doctor tells them their thyroid test is normal. Any number of books are available on the subject, but my favorites are *Hypothyroidism: The Unsuspected Illness* (Harper and Row 1976), by Dr. Broda O. Barnes and Lawrence Calton, and *Living Well with Hypothyroidism* (2000), by Mary Shomon. Both of these books tell the story of people devastated by inaccurate lab tests and doctors who don't understand the tests. The tests themselves are not at fault. But the practitioners who have a patient in front of them with all the clinical signs of a disease and who will defer in their judgment to a test are missing the diagnosis.

It turns out there are a number of conditions that may lead to normal thyroid test results in persons with low functioning thyroid glands. Not so ironic is that one of these conditions, autoimmune disease of the thyroid, represents an abnormal immune response not unlike food sensitivities. The immune system has long baffled the experts. In lieu of searching for and understanding the underlying cause of immune disease, most immunology specialists are content to prescribe medication or the very lucrative allergy shots. Many doctors have seen a clear link between food intolerance, causing gastrointestinal disturbance and then autoimmune mediated thyroid disease.

At any rate, thyroid disease from any cause may result in lowered metabolism. Thus the tired, cold feeling. Under the direction of a low-functioning thyroid, it is very difficult to keep from gaining weight. And if one has food sensitivities accompanying the low thyroid function, as often happens, a desolate spiral of weight gain, depression, and fatigue are imminent. Often in the prime of life after having a child, women find themselves abandoned by a medical system that does not acknowledge their thyroid disease and/or food sensitivities.

Serotonin and the ALCAT Test

This chapter offers a brief glimpse of what's involved in the complex area of obesity and biochemistry. The exact roles of the many neurotransmitters and hormones involved in obesity are not yet clear and require further research. But based on current theories and preliminary research, we can make an educated guess that the effect of food intolerance on these powerful biochemical and genetic forces is significant. Take serotonin, for example, which controls how we feel: If we eat certain carbohydrates, serotonin levels increase and we feel better. Serotonin is a chemical substance primarily present in the white blood cells and platelets—the very cells that change because of the presence of allergenic foods. This change is what the ALCAT test measures.

Research already conducted on the ALCAT test shows that people who stop eating foods to which they are intolerant find that among other things, their "craving for sweets" is diminished.

Research already conducted on the ALCAT test shows that people who stop eating foods to which they are intolerant find that among other things, their "craving for sweets" is diminished. This strongly suggests that food intolerances somehow impact serotonin functioning. In fact, one study on food allergy mediators conducted in Australia and reported by Dr. Colin H. Little in *Food Allergy and Intolerance* (1987), edited by Drs. Jonathan Brostoff and Stephen J. Challacombe, shows that eating an allergenic food often lowers the blood levels of serotonin. Lower levels of serotonin make you uncomfortable, and you turn to simple sugars and carbohydrates for relief. Eating highly refined carbohydrates and sugars triggers a rapid release of insulin, which in turn reduces concentrations of all amino acids in the blood, except for tryptophan, a precursor of serotonin. Timothy D. Brewerston, M.D., writes in the May 1986 *Nutrition Reviews Supplement,*

"The appetite, affective and impulsive features of bulimia have all been associated with possible alterations in serotonin transmission."

Thus, to compensate for lower brain levels of serotonin, caused by eating the offending foods, food-sensitive people tend to crave foods that increase serotonin in the brain. According to nutrition researcher, Judith J. Wurtman, Ph.D., from M.I.T., "Serotonin is the calming chemical. When the brain is using it, feelings of stress and tension are eased." ("Sweet Relief With On-the-Spot Tranquilizers," *Prevention*, Sept. 1988). This sets up a vicious cycle of food cravings and addiction. Medical science would bring in a drug at this point to temporarily relieve this craving, but research on food intolerance shows that you can get a permanent, non-pharmaceutical effect by removing the allergenic foods that trigger the serotonin imbalance in the first place.

ALCAT: The Bottom Line

As already noted, research on the ALCAT test shows that people who stop eating foods they do not tolerate well find that their "craving for sweets" is diminished. This strongly suggests that the intolerant foods, which damaged the white blood cells, also disrupted the chemicals in those cells, thus continuing the patient's cycles of obesity and poor health.

The bottom line is that all the drawbacks of conventional weight loss diets are removed when people follow diets that remove foods they do not tolerate as identified by the ALCAT test. In the next few chapters, we'll explore the connection between weight loss and food intolerance, and illustrate how the ALCAT test helps people identify their food intolerances and find their way back to their ideal weight.

Synopsis

1. Fat is necessary for life, and our ability to store fat is working against us.

2. Lifestyle, processed foods, environmental chemicals, and lack of exercise contribute to weight gain.

3. The multibillion-dollar commercial weight loss industry thrives because it doesn't deliver weight loss.

4. Diet drugs have very limited value unless the underlying cause of weight gain is addressed.

5. Several biochemical forces come into play as weight gain progresses.

6. The ALCAT test identifies foods that contribute to weight gain.

CHAPTER 3

Breakthrough Research on Obesity and Health

At current rates, every single person in the United States will be obese by the year 2230.

—from research conducted by
World Health Organization (WHO) task force, May 1996

The number of Americans with diabetes has jumped nearly 50 percent since 1983 and tripled since the late 1950s.

—from a 1995 study by the National Institute of Diabetes

Overweight and obesity may not be infectious diseases, but they have reached epidemic proportions in the United States.

—U.S. Surgeon General, 2001

In 1999 an estimated 61 percent of U.S. adults were over-weight or obese, and 13 percent of children and adolescents were overweight.

—U.S. Surgeon General's report, December 2001

The four statistics just given are just some of the many alarming reports on the state of our health as we enter the 21st century. These statistics should surprise anyone familiar with the amazing advances that took place in the field of medicine in the 20th century. One hundred years ago doctors could do little more than set broken bones, lance boils, and soothe symptoms; they could seldom cure disease. By the middle of the century all that had changed. Medical science began making breathtaking advances, and medicine began triumphing over many health problems such as infectious diseases, heart disease, some cancers, brain disease, and immune system malfunctions, to name a few.

And yet, as we exit this amazing century in medicine and enter the 21st century, medical science is still battling some common illnesses that cripple and kill millions of people around the world. Not only are we seemingly losing ground on some health problems that have been around for decades, but we're also facing a growing number of new problems.

This predicament forces the question—what exactly is going on? The United States has the greatest medical science in the world, yet a good deal of today's research points to one shocking fact—as a whole, we're getting fatter and sicker. Clearly, part of the medical puzzle is still missing— and that missing piece is keeping too many of us and our children from the optimal health we all desire. This situation does not result from a lack of effort to find solutions; it may instead result from looking for answers in the wrong places or looking at our health from the wrong perspective.

Medical science has no shortage of new treatments and new research underway for ever-new understanding of the human body, the nature of specific diseases, and cures for those diseases. Every day, in popular magazines, daily newspapers, and television and radio reports, we hear about the latest medical treatments and research.

For example, obesity has recently been cited as the second biggest health concern of our age. Indeed, this is no small health problem: Obesity alone accounts for the overwhelming increase in diabetes, heart disease, and high blood pressure. An immense amount of groundbreaking research is currently underway in the worldwide effort to find a solution to this nearly out-of-control medical problem. Today drug therapy, gene manipulation, hormonal activity, and other biochemical functions are currently under intense scrutiny in laboratories around the world-researchers are conducting hundreds of studies in their search for a way to end what's been called "the plague of our age."

New Hope for the Overweight

All this research on obesity sounds exciting and full of potential, but within the mountains of study conclusions, few offer definitive solutions. The prognosis for a life of ideal weight is still grim into the foreseeable future.

In the middle of this storm of speculation and disappointment, one obesity and health research study was quietly conducted in 1995 at Columbia/HCA Medical Center's Sports Medicine and Performance Center in Houston and at Baylor Medical College. One hundred overweight patients who had at least two other health problems, such as migraines and chronic tiredness, were studied. This four-week trial, which studied the impact of food intolerance on obesity and other common health problems, led to extraordinary results.

The 50 study participants who eliminated foods identified by a simple blood test measuring adverse reactions in their bodies lost not just body weight but body fat. In fact, these subjects lost an average of nearly 3 pounds of fat and gained almost 1 pound of lean muscle. The 50 "control" subjects, on the other hand, who followed their own weight loss plans, gained an average of 1 pound of fat and lost almost 1 pound of lean muscle. Overall, the two groups' body composition (lean-to-fat ratio) showed a 6-pound difference at the end of the four-week trial. Calculated from a statistical perspective, these differences are highly significant.

The United States has the greatest medical science in the world, yet a good deal of today's research points to one shocking fact—as a whole, we're getting fatter and sicker.

Still more astounding, the participants in the experimental group improved significantly and dramatically in 20 of 24 disease symptoms when compared to their counterparts who followed dietary plans of their own choosing. This 1996 study achieved results—measurable changes in body weight, body composition, and disease symptoms with a simple, nonpharmaceutical therapy. "We found that you can change people's health dramatically when you remove their intolerant foods from their diets," noted the principal investigator of the study, Gilbert Kaats, Ph.D. Dr. Kaats, who is the director of the Health and Medical Research Foundation, an independent research organization in San

Antonio, Texas, added that "[determining] food intolerance is extremely helpful in improving health and losing weight. It's much more effective than traditional dieting."

Common Foods Can
Sabotage Your Health

Dr. Kaats's breakthrough study demonstrated a remarkable and unprecedented occurrence within the bodies of the 50 "experimenters" (as they're called in research parlance) who eliminated the respective foods to which each was shown to be biochemically sensitive. What occurred? By not eating the foods they could not tolerate, the 50 "experimenters" eliminated substances that disrupted their body's immune system, brain chemistry, and/or digestive system.

These findings are among the first to support a theory that a growing number of medical doctors have held for decades: By eliminating reactive or allergenic foods from a person's diet, you remove the substances that trigger the health problems in the first place. These foods have been exacerbating the problems through repeated exposure.

For example, the immune system may have overreacted to what it perceived as an "invader" (the intolerant food or a chemical in the food), which it then attacked, just as it would attack a virus or a bacteria. Or the reactive foods may have caused the body's sensitive brain chemistry to go haywire, creating food cravings that triggered eating binges or disrupted metabolism. Or they compounded digestive system deficiencies, resulting in malabsorption that exacerbated the obesity and health problems. Once one or more of these reactions begins, the body's systems are no longer able to operate at optimum performance levels.

Once their troublemaking foods were out of the way, the research participants' immune systems, brain chemistry, and digestive systems were no longer struggling to operate under adverse conditions. Instead, they adjusted to the healthier internal "climate" and functioned at maximum performance—metabolizing the safe foods more effectively, burning stored fat more efficiently, neutralizing food cravings, eliminating water retention, and clearing away health symptoms. "Our findings are consistent with the latest biochemical and genetic research," Dr. Kaats adds. "It looks like when some people eat certain foods, which could be anything from milk products to lettuce, they experience an allergic-like reaction. With regards to weight loss, instead of getting a rash or going into anaphylactic shock, their appetite and food cravings increase. Eliminating these allergenic foods appears to balance appetite, food cravings, and body composition."

The World That Technology Built

Exactly what do the current statistics on the state of our health at the turn of this century say about our sophisticated medical technology? And what do the results of this small research study, which took such a simple step to correct health problems and got such dramatic results, say about treating today's mounting health care problems?

You can find answers to these questions by looking back a hundred years ago, before medical science and medical technology transformed the world by creating cures and treatments for many of the ills of the human body. As medical science began to take off in the early 1900s, it naturally focused on the health care epidemics of the time—tuberculosis, bacterial infections, scarlet fever, and smallpox, to name a few. By mid-century, as research moved us toward greater technological advances in heart, brain, and cancer treatments, for example, it took a definitive turn that shaped the "traditional" medical treatment we receive today, including the development of potent pharmaceuticals.

In the race to find treatments and cures for the ailments of the 19th century, medical science appears to have had one major shortcoming—it could not keep up with the problems that were developing, ironically, as a result of 20th-century technology. (In all fairness, nobody had a crystal ball that allowed him or her to peer into the future and see what troubles were brewing.) The outcome was that researchers and doctors, by and large, were not able to address the "new" health problems. These problems were being created and compounded by the very developments in medical science that were supposed to eradicate health problems in our lifetimes. Technological developments in other industries further exacerbated the health threat to 20th-century Americans. As it was, medical science was not the only industry making giant leaps forward in technology.

With the 20th century behind us, we can look back and see clearly how our world changed in a hundred years. For example, whereas our forefathers traveled by horse and buggy, we travel by car, train, and plane. Whereas a century ago all farming was "organic," today each of us consumes pounds of chemicals each year, all added as we grow, transport, package, and cook our food. And while people at the turn of the 20th century lived slow-paced lives close to home, today we travel daily to offices miles from home, sit in rush-hour traffic, and largely communicate with each other by such impersonal modes as phone, fax, and e-mail. No one would argue that in a hundred years we've created a very different world.

The net result of such changes is that while doctors around the world advanced from mere lancing of boils and setting of bones to performing incredible medical miracles, our world was becoming increasingly adulterated. The amazing technological advances that have changed our planet more in the last hundred years than in the entire previous history of the human race, have also brought a slew of environmental health hazards in the form of air pollution, water pollution, and heavily adulterated and nutritionally deficient foods. In the final analysis, this downside to progress may well be the core of many, if not all, of today's mounting health care problems. Ironically, as technology has become more sophisticated, aimed toward making our lives better, it has placed our bodies in a relatively unnatural environment—both internally and externally.

A High-Tech Solution to Health Care

Clearly, we now need health care that takes into account the world that 20th-century technology has created. We must find the missing puzzle piece that will stop diseases such as obesity, diabetes, cardiovascular disease, asthma, ear infections, attention deficit disorder, and other health problems from running rampant. This elusive piece may not be a miracle drug or expensive surgical procedure; it may be as simple as removing the foods that contribute to the 20th-century overload with which our bodies contend daily.

Luckily, along with other high-tech developments in medical science, a simple test has been invented that easily and quickly analyzes blood cells to determine the exact foods, food chemicals, and other substances to which a person is intolerant. Although many medical practitioners (called "environmental physicians") used the food intolerance concept to treat patients in previous decades, they could only help a limited number of people because testing was a slow, tedious, often uncomfortable process.

This research on health and obesity and other studies on food intolerance using the new blood-testing procedure have led researchers to discover that the simple step of removing foods to which one is intolerant brings permanent relief from often chronic health care problems that no medicine or procedure previously could resolve. Others have benefited from overall changes in how they live their lives and treat their bodies. To make significant strides in medicine in the 21st century, we need to address the real world of chemicals, pollution, and modern stressors. And to effectively do that, we must add food intolerance testing to the physician's bag of great medical treatments available today.

Food Intolerance:
Breakthrough Diagnosis and Treatment

Have you ever gone to a doctor and complained of a headache, tiredness, an upset stomach, or some other persistent condition? If so, what did the doctor say? "Take two aspirin" or "Get more sleep." Maybe he or she did some test and then said, "Nothing's wrong, it must all be in your head." Or quite possibly the doctor simply gave you a prescription for some drug. If you or someone you know has experienced such medical treatment, you're not alone. Thousands of people receive this diagnosis every day in medical offices across America. Is it any wonder that most people do not share such chronic, low-grade symptoms with their physicians?

What about the last weight loss diet you went on? Did it leave you feeling hungry, low on energy, cranky and nervous, or craving particular foods like sweets? Then, after all the trouble of counting calories, cutting back on fats, and feeling awful, did you finally give in, binge on the foods you craved, and gain back the weight you lost? This is the sad story for millions of dieters across the country every day. They eat salads, drink skim milk, and sip bottled water, at least until they can't take it anymore and devour a donut or consume a bag of chips in 30 seconds flat. Then they start thinking about how they can get their hands on the next food they crave. This is a troubling, stressful life for our powerful, yet delicate bodies. It's no wonder that as a nation we're fatter than ever.

Or perhaps you're the parent of a child with chronic ear infections, or one who's been labeled with attention deficit hyperactivity disorder (ADHD). Maybe your child's chronic headaches and stomachaches cost you precious hours visiting the doctor's office, taking time off from work, or lying awake at night? Do doctors recommend surgery to insert ear tubes or prescription drugs like Ritalin to deal with your child's health problems? If so, you have a lot of company. Today, there is a literal epidemic of children diagnosed with otitis media (ear infections) and ADHD—and the traditional medical treatments for these two conditions are surgery and drugs. What message do we give our children about their health care now and in the future?

The Modern World
Confounds Traditional Medicine

If any of the situations just mentioned remind you of your experiences or those of someone you know, welcome to traditional modern medicine. It's a world of surgery and prescription drugs, and little else. And it's guided by an impersonal, efficient philosophy that focuses on treating the symptoms rather than the sources of health problems. Meanwhile, the modern world is full of stress, pollution, and preservative-filled, chemically packed, and genetically altered "food." And it appears certain that the situation will continue.

But do these factors play a part in the medicine doctors practice on our bodies? The sad answer is, not often. One study, for example, found that less than 4 percent of the population gets its nutritional information from doctors. Interestingly, the same study, conducted by the American Dietetic Association for its 1995 Nutritional Trends Survey, reported that 39 percent of the population say they get most of their nutritional information from magazines.

For all the billions spent on medical care, we have seen surprisingly little progress in combating major and minor diseases.

Meanwhile, medical companies give the illusion of accomplishing great things in these same magazines. You can hardly pick up a newspaper or magazine without reading an advertisement or article for another "breakthrough drug" to treat arthritis, depression, weight loss, asthma, or any of a long list of common medical problems. What's more, billions of dollars go into research to develop pharmaceuticals, therapies, and medical equipment to treat our ailments. We have access to all these phenomenal medical accomplishments, yet as a nation are sicker and fatter than ever. In fact, for all the billions spent on medical care, we have seen surprisingly little progress in combating major and minor diseases.

Look at any illness—including diabetes, arthritis, asthma, cancer, and obesity—and you'll find that it's on the rise instead of the decline. Yet when you see advertisements for the latest drugs and therapies, you'd expect everyone to be brimming with health—all we have to do is take those magic pills. Something is wrong with this picture. Modern medicine focuses largely on treating symptoms, and all but ignores the sources of our mounting health ills.

More than one critic has expressed concern for the current state of our health care system. For example, in his book *Dear America, a Concerned Doctor Wants You to Know the Truth about Health Reform,* published in 1993, Melvin Konner, M.D., wrote,

> What has happened to American medicine's Golden Age? Just a couple of decades ago it seemed as though doctors could do no wrong. Medical miracles lay like jewels to be picked up each time we turned a corner. Penicillin, streptomycin, cortisone, polio vaccine, open-heart surgery, the heart-lung machine, psychiatric drugs, kidney dialysis, transplants—three decades ago there seemed to be no end to what we could do, and no limit to medicine's confidence. America clearly did have the best health care in the world, and it seemed sure only to get better. Yet today there is widespread agreement that the system is not working.

Our health care is now to the point that we have to ask ourselves: Are these expensive, high-tech therapies helping or are they hurting our health?

The summer 1995 edition of *Health & Wellness Today,* published by Julian Whitaker, M.D., comments,

• Doctors get free vacations, computers, cellular phones, even free educations for prescribing certain drugs— whether or not they are good for you!

- In a major study, Boston University researchers found that 36 percent of hospital admissions are caused by doctors' blunders! . . .

- A seven-year study of 90,000 women, ages 40–59, showed that those who had regular mammograms were subjected to twice the surgical procedures and more mastectomies than those who didn't—yet life expectancy is exactly the same! Mastectomies were used for over a hundred years before anyone did a study to see if they were effective (they weren't).

- According to the *New England Journal of Medicine,* balloon angioplasty—a $4 billion-per-year business—kills 9,000 people a year . . . even though there's never been a study to prove it does any good! Heart bypass operations—a $10 million-per-day industry kill 28,000 Americans every year, even though two big studies have proven bypass surgery does not make patients live longer!

- Even doctors admit that 900,000 unnecessary angiograms are done every year in the United States alone. And 4,500 people die needlessly as a result!

- Each year, two million patients pick up hospital infections that they didn't have before they were admitted. Of those, about 60,000 die from the infection.

So, if the way doctors are practicing medicine today isn't working, what then is the way to achieve the optimum health that we all desire and deserve?

The Environmental Epidemic
of the 21st Century

When, if ever, will our health care system take into account the mounting attacks our bodies have to deal with in today's world—pollution, stress, and food chemicals. Pollution has been a growing health problem for decades and has even been linked to death. An environmental advocacy group, the Natural Resources Defense Council, released a report in early 1996 linking certain types of air pollution—from combustion of coal, oil, gas, diesel, and wood, and high-temperature processing such as copper smelting and steel mills—to the premature deaths of about 64,000 Americans a year.

Stress has been a known detriment to poor health for decades—yet our society only encourages more and more stress-producing lifestyles. Stress has been associated with vitamin, mineral, and amino acid depletion. This depleted store of nutrients leads to mood swings, anger and rage, depression, insomnia, food cravings, anxiety, and panic attacks. Food sensitivities or allergies are in themselves stress to the body. Take a "normal" run of the mill stressful day and add to it a nutrient weak fast food diet, throw a little sugar and food sensitivities in and you have a catastrophe waiting to happen. Stress is difficult to manage or treat without close attention to diet. One must slow the depletion of nutrients while replacing them with either supplements or a carefully chosen diet. Slow the depletion of nutrients by avoiding sugars, processed grains, and stop eating the foods you are sensitive to.

Then there is the problem of increasing chemicals and genetically engineered food. In fact, Drs. Claudia. Miller and Nicolas Ashford, in their book *Chemical Exposures* (1991), allege that each year every adult in the United States consumes 24 pounds of synthetic chemicals.

Given these challenging conditions—and they are just the tip of the iceberg—is it any wonder that food intolerance is growing more prevalent, as many specialists suggest? Indeed, it may even be, as many predict, the epidemic of the new century. Estimates on the prevalence of food intolerance range from 30 to 90 percent of the population suffering from some degree of the condition. Perhaps food intolerance is a sign that the human body has not fully adapted to the novel environment we have created for ourselves. Is this the legacy we want to pass on to our children in the 21st century?

The Cost of Bad Health
and Poor Health Care

Many are profiting from our ill health—drug companies, diet product companies, developers of expensive medical technologies, makers of convenience foods—and the list goes on. Everyone, it seems, is profiting but us. The American health care system is among the biggest profit enterprises in the country. In 1992, according to the U.S. Commerce Department, Americans spent $847 billion on health care. By 1995, the cost of treating disease had reached in excess of $1 trillion. By the year 2000, health care costs reached an astonishing $1.3 trillion.

It's nearly impossible to determine the amount of money spent on any given disease; too many factors must be considered. But one thing is certain: It's costing more every year to treat any given disease. Take a look at just one of today's most common diseases: diabetes. Of the 8 million Americans diagnosed with diabetes (it's believed that another 8 million are undiagnosed), direct medical costs per year in the United States are $45 billion, while the indirect cost from disability is approaching another $47 billion, according to the National Institutes of Health.

Pharmaceutical companies, each of which has a large advertising budget, are among the most profitable corporations. They produce a large variety of increasingly more expensive drugs, and they profit however they can. Drug companies' attempts to further increase their profits through underhanded measures are the subject of many reports.

One such report appeared in the *Wall Street Journal* on April 25, 1996. The article tells how one of the biggest drug companies paid a university to conduct a study on a new drug for hypothyroidism, a metabolic disorder that affects a diagnosed 8 million Americans. Then the drug company undermined the results because the study found the new drug was virtually identical to three cheaper versions. The study also found that U.S. health care costs could be cut by $356 million a year if the new drugs were replaced by the cheaper, but equally effective, drugs. When one hears stories like this, it's easy to understand why people are often disillusioned with 21st-century medicine.

Time for a New Medical Paradigm

What if medicine were practiced differently? What if the whole body were taken into consideration when a patient presented a chronic complaint? What if stress, pollution, and the foods we eat day in and day out were considered in our overall health? What if treatment of food intolerance were considered a viable route to good health? Surely, medicine would take a big turn for the better. It's difficult to precisely analyze the cost savings if a person were to prevent a disease from developing in the first place. But it's easy to imagine incredible savings if millions of people did not acquire diabetes, arthritis, obesity, gastrointestinal problems, and a host of other common illnesses, thereby avoiding untold years of doctor visits, drug therapies, surgeries, and time off work.

Here's what a few of today's experts in food intolerance have to say about this therapy:

> The scientific investigations increasingly point toward the importance of applying food intolerance testing to patients' overall health care. It's extremely important that practitioners

put action behind their words, and do more to both prevent and treat this popular disease.

—Dr. Lene Høj, an internal medical doctor and specialist
in allergic diseases who operates a large private practice
in Copenhagen, Denmark

If food intolerance treatments were widely used, we'd see many more chronic conditions improve, including depression, mood swings, and overweight.

—Dr. John Magauran, a general practitioner
in private practice in Honolulu, Hawaii

I think that it's underestimated how many problems are related to food intolerance.

—Dr. Jay Sandweiss, an internal medicine practitioner
specializing in environmental medicine in Detroit

The possibility that diet may play a significant role in some patients and the usually benign nature of investigation required make it worthwhile to attempt to answer this question in any chronic disorder which is otherwise not adequately treatable or in which the usual prescribed treatment carries with it some hazard or adverse effect.

—Dr. Douglas H. Sandberg, formerly director of the
Department of Pediatrics, Division of Gastroenterology
and Nutrition, in the Allergic and Environmental Disease Unit
at the University of Miami Children's Hospital Center in Miami

I've had a great deal of satisfaction treating diet-related problems, for by doing so one gets to the root of the problem, and away from simply dishing out medications which treat symptoms, and provide only symptomatic relief.

—Dr. John W. Gerrard, an allergy and immunology specialist
and former professor of pediatrics at the
University of Saskatchewan in Saskatchewan, Canada

Most of the people I see have three common problems—fatigue, depression, and difficulty with concentration, which they don't even mention until after they've eliminated their intolerant foods and those symptoms clear up. Many patients have told me, "I've had those symptoms for years and now they're gone." That's nice to hear.

—Dr. Richard Bahr, an environmental medicine specialist
in private practice in Cincinnati

With any other traditional therapy you have side effects, whereas with food intolerance testing there is no down side, and there is an absolute up side.

—Dr. David Cafarelli, a medical practitioner
specializing in nutrition in West Palm Beach

Food Intolerance Testing to the Rescue

It's time we actually did live our day-to-day lives with the vim and vigor portrayed in magazine advertisements. It's time we lived free from unnecessary chronic health complaints. And it's time we lived life to the fullest instead of being needlessly weighted down by poor health and obesity. By addressing food intolerance, thousands of people already made this goal a reality because they took a step that is rarely mentioned in traditional medicine—they removed the cause of their health complaints, instead of just masking the symptoms with a drug or other medical treatment. Many have already found that the cure for their health problems, whether minor or severe, was as simple as removing foods that, for one reason or another, did not agree with their systems.

If food intolerance is so widespread, why, you may wonder, haven't you heard about it until now? That's a good question. And the answer is firmly rooted in the fact that food intolerance does not, for some reason, fit into the modern, "traditional" model of medicine. Many doctors simply do not accept it as a viable medical condition.

The seed of this thinking begins in medical school, where the human body is broken into pieces to be studied and treated. As a result, if you have a sore throat you go to an ear, nose, and throat specialist; if you have a stomach problem you go to a gastroenterologist; and if you have a yeast infection you go to a gynecologist. This medical paradigm leaves little room for a treatment that requires a doctor to acknowledge that what a person puts in his or her mouth may cause a pain in his head, an infection in her ear, or itchy skin in the groin. Many doctors who practice what's called "alternative" medicine have broken out of the traditional mold and taken a different path—either because of a personal health experience or because they took a critical look at traditional medicine and didn't like what they saw.

For all the billions spent on medical care, we have seen surprisingly little progress in combating major and minor diseases. Ironically, Hippocrates himself, the "father of medicine," said 2,500 years ago,

> It appears to me necessary to every physician to be skilled in nature, and to strive to know, if he would wish to perform his duties, what man is in relation to the articles of food and drink, and to his occupations, and what are the effects of each of them to every one.

Yet today, as mentioned, food and nutrition are rarely discussed in the thousands of doctors' offices across the country.

Prescription Drugs: Just Say "No"?

Medical treatment typically consists of giving a chemical to relieve, cover up, or resolve a disease process, while the principal treatment of food intolerance consists of removing the offending agent. By disconnecting the parts of the body, medical practitioners disregard the impact one part of the body may have on another, which leads to another major aspect of medicine today—prescription drugs. If you're treating a disease as an entity, separate from all other functions of the body, then why not simply zap it with a drug? Never mind the short- and long-term side effects that drug may have on other organs of the body. Right now, in the short term, you're successful at relieving the migraine, infection, joint pain, ADHD, or weight problem.

Antibiotics alone, although powerful drugs that have saved many lives, also contribute to many health problems. Earlier this century, breakthroughs in antibiotics inspired confident predictions that all kinds of modern-day illnesses would be eradicated. But antibiotics have a sinister side—an adverse effect on the intestinal wall. The small intestine is host not just to unfriendly bacteria, but also to the friendly bacteria that we need to keep our digestive system healthy. Antibiotics act like a Hoover, vacuuming out all bacteria, whether unfriendly or friendly. Because antibiotics have been overused since they were introduced in the 1930s, many of us are faced with the consequences—chronic illness.

Another factor facing modern health care is wave after wave of newly drug-resistant microbes; and we are running out of antibiotics to fight them. Just one example of this problem is illustrated in the preliminary findings of a two-year study, conducted at the University of Texas, on the use of antibiotics to treat chronic ear infections. The study found that more and more doctors were seeing children with ear infections who didn't respond to first-line antibiotic treatments (as many as 50 percent). This was forcing the doctors to resort to stronger drugs that cause diarrhea and upset stomachs. This problem has developed because bacteria have an incredible ability to become resistant to antibiotics.

Is the Cure Worse
Than the Disease?

Despite the inconveniences, prescription drugs won't lose their luster any time soon. For one thing, drugs are a quick treatment. A doctor can write a prescription in 30 seconds, whereas discussing nutrition and other preventative health care concerns could take hours. Clearly, by prescribing drugs, a physician can see more patients per day and have a more profitable practice. Of course, prescription drugs have their place in medicine; few medical practitioners would dispute that fact. But a growing number of medical practitioners and patient advocacy groups suspect that the prescription drug trend is getting out of control— to the detriment of the health it's designed to improve.

On this note, John Braithwaite made an interesting observation in his book *Corporate Crime in the Pharmaceutical Industry* (1984). He pointed out in a chapter entitled "The Corporation as Pusher" that:

> People who foster dependence on illicit drugs such as
> heroin are regarded as among the most unscrupulous pariahs of modern civilization. In contrast, pushers of licit drugs
> tend to be viewed as altruistically motivated purveyors of a
> social good. Yet dependence on Valium or Darvon can have
> consequences just as frightening as heroin addiction.

On this note, it's important to mention the perhaps most overused medication "pushed" on a frighteningly high number of our children—Ritalin. This amphetamine-like agent is standard therapy for hyperactive children, despite the fact that this drug is addictive and can cause psychotic behavior. In fact, Ritalin is one of the most popular forms of "speed" in the drug culture, drawing high prices in the illicit drug trafficking trade. Furthermore, Dr. Sidney Wolfe, head of a respected Washington public interest group that, among other things, evaluates drugs for consumers, pointed out in the early 1990s that 104 of the 287 most frequently prescribed drugs are too dangerous to use.

Prescription drugs are not the only medicines that may be undermining the health of many people. More than one study has found that over-the-counter medications may be more harmful than people realize. Case after case deals with people who took common pain relievers, asthma medications, cough and cold medicines, or nasal sprays and suffered joint pain, headaches, swollen blood vessels, indigestion, heartburn, liver damage, even death. Often doctors and the FDA blame the people themselves for using the medications incorrectly. But the fact is that most medication that has a good effect in one part of your body also has a negative side effect, usually on some other part of the body.

Aspirin, for example, one of the most common drugs used today, has a wide range of actions and a long list of beneficial effects, but also has one or two drawbacks. Every aspirin a person takes will slightly damage the intestinal wall and lead to a small amount of bleeding. The higher the dose, the greater the bleeding and damage. It's been found that a weakened gut wall, the only barrier between the body's digestion and elimination system and the bloodstream, can lead to severe health problems, including food intolerance. This is not the side effect people need when they take a small pill to get rid of a headache or joint pain. It's like taking one step forward and two steps back in our race to achieve long-term maximum health.

Walking the High Road to Wellness

Clearly, it's time we take a serious look at the way health care is practiced today so we can direct it down a more successful path tomorrow. And it's time we bring the successful, so-called alternative treatment of food intolerance out of the shadows and give many who suffer from poor health a chance to live free of disease. Consider this: Some medical practitioners estimate that 90 to 95 percent of all chronic illnesses are preventable. One of the easiest ways to keep people healthy is to avoid sickness or detect illness early.

But implementing this philosophy will require a paradigm shift in the thinking of our traditional medical practitioners, and in that of the insurance companies and HMOs that now control access to health care. Because HMOs profit by keeping sick people out of the system, this philosophy should fit in well with their business plans. By taking an active role in promoting good health, giving people access to the health care services and tools, such as diagnostic tests, HMOs can ensure maximum health— clearly a win-win situation for both the companies and their patients.

Synopsis

1. Independent and medical school collaborated studies confirm the benefits of ALCAT food sensitivity testing.
2. Identifying reactive foods eliminates many of the unpleasant effects of dieting.
3. Traditional medicine is slow to accept food sensitivity science that is not promoted by large drug companies.
4. Open-minded doctors are realizing the benefits of testing for food sensitivities.
5. Overuse and misuse of prescription medication contributes to health care miseries.

CHAPTER 4

A Short Course in the Science of Food Intolerance

The body's immune system includes teams of specialized cells, some of which contain arsenals of powerful chemicals. These cells are like loyal and eager troops of foot soldiers, awaiting instructions from their commanding officers, prepared to defend the body from foreign invaders at a moment's notice. They are armed with chemicals such as histamine and other preformed mediators—typically inactive, but always awaiting the signal that will cause their release. Enter an unfriendly bacteria, virus, parasite, or any foreign substance that the immune system believes might be harmful, and immune cells are brought to attention, prepared to release their chemical weapons to fight the invader.

The Role of the Immune System

The immune system not only surveys the body for precancerous and cancerous cells, but it also eliminates debris;

and, as mentioned earlier, it must protect the body against attack from a variety of harmful pathogens. It must do so while discriminating between what is harmful and what is not harmful. It must also not attack any of the body's own healthy tissue. Thus it has evolved a broad repertoire of responses to deal with the various situations it encounters.

An outburst of destructive chemicals is one of the many actions that keep us safe. Although the immune system comprises a sophisticated mechanism of self-defense, literally fighting enemies around the clock, occasionally a glitch occurs; for example, when the body develops an allergy to an otherwise harmless substance, such as a peanut or cat dander. Thus the same powerful chemical response that is usually directed toward foreign pathogens, such as bacteria, viruses, and parasites, can react as powerfully against an innocuous substance, one that is harmless to most individuals. This is clearly one instance in which the "cure" is worse than the disease. The severity of reactions varies from mild and barely noticeable to life threatening, such as when a person goes into anaphylactic shock, causing serious illness and possibly death.

The immune response can also be directed against its own tissue, a sort of "friendly fire" phenomenon, causing an autoimmune disorder. These disorders include multiple sclerosis, thyroid conditions, lupus, rheumatoid arthritis, scleraderma, and others. Food intolerance can be the cause of this. Dr. Loren Cordain, author of *The Paleo Diet,* explains, "All autoimmune diseases develop because of interactions between the genes and one or more environmental factors, such as a viral or bacterial infection or exposure to certain food. . . . Surprisingly, we have found that many common gut bacteria fragments are made up of the same molecular building blocks as those found in certain immune system proteins and in some of the tissues under attack by the immune system. This three-way matchup—of gut bacteria or food protein, immune system protein, and body tissue protein—may confuse the immune system, causing it to attack the body's own tissue."

Yet we cannot even survive for even one day without the immune system, as seen from the well-known case of the child who came to be known as the "bubble boy" because, literally, he had to live within a plastic bubble to protect him from any and all the pathogens in the air. A level of pathogen that a normal immune system neutralizes automatically, without the owner of the immune system even taking notice, would be deadly to someone with *SCIDS*—severe combined immune deficiency, caused, in part, when the genes do not encode for a critical enzyme called adenosine deaminase.

We can also acquire immune deficiency, from lifestyle and/or infection, as in acquired immune deficiency syndrome (AIDS), which renders one prone to all kinds of opportunistic infections and cancers. However it happens, if the immune system fails, we cannot survive.

There are other disorders mediated by the immune system. It is also the immune system that causes the damage to heart tissue following a heart attack. The "attack" is caused by a temporary stoppage of blood flow occurring when a clot obstructs an already narrowed artery. The greatest damage actually occurs when the blood flow to the heart tissue resumes, a process called reperfusion. Certain phagocytic white blood cells, called neutrophils, release inflammatory chemical mediators that attack the heart tissue itself, thus causing the damage.

Juvenile diabetes (as distinguished from adult onset or Type 2 diabetes) is another disease brought about when the same white cells of the immune system, primarily the nutrophils, attack the insulin-producing cells in the pancreas. Also, the damage to the liver associated with hepatitis C infection is the collateral damage caused by the immune system cells attacking the virus in the liver.

How is this collateral damage caused? As mentioned, once activated a subclass of immune system cells, which includes phagocytes, releases powerful chemicals, chemicals not only capable of causing fatal damage to foreign invaders, such as pathogenic bacteria; but also capable, when misdirected, of causing damage to the host. These chemicals wreak their destructive force because they contain free radicals. Free radicals (not to be confused with political activists on the loose) also known as reactive oxygen specials, are of different types. They can be highly destructive. Any molecule can become a free radical by either gaining or losing an electron from its orbit. The atom then seeks to re-establish its own equilibrium by stealing electrons from neighboring atoms. Once this movement is initiated, these molecules set up a cascade reaction.

Professor emeritus of immunology (University of California at Los Angeles) William R. Clark, in his 1999 book *A Means to an End: the Biological Basis of Aging,* explains the process by which cells of the innate immune system inflict damage on potential pathogens. The innate immune system, as opposed to the adaptive or specific immune system, includes not only the body's natural barriers, protective antibodies and special proteins in the blood that attack bacteria (called the complement system) but also the phagocytic immune cells. The general protective function of this branch of the immune system is regarded as the primary line of defense against harmful foreign micro-organisms and substances.

What we see is that the immune system is really a double-edged sword: protective when operating appropriately, and damaging to the host when overly or inappropriately active. Clark writes,

> One of the more common sources of reactive oxygen species in the body as a whole is from cells that use the destructive power of these molecules as a natural defense against microbial infection. Phagocytes (literally, "eaters of cells") such as

macrophages and neutrophils purposely generate high levels of oxygen radicals, which they store in tightly sealed intracellular compartments. When phagocytes engulf bacteria or other microbes during the course of an infection, they deliver them from these internal radical-containing compartments, where they are very efficiently destroyed. Unfortunately, after several rounds of microbial feeding, the phagocytes die and release their contents into the surrounding tissues. Oxygen radicals released in this fashion can be taken up by adjacent cells, and once inside they cause the same sort of damage as radicals produced internally. . . . [I]n the case of prolonged infections a chronic inflammatory state may develop, and the repeated engorging and death of phagocytes can cause serious oxidative damage to nearby healthy cells. This is also a major source of damage in chronic inflammatory autoimmune reactions such as rheumatoid arthritis, and can lead to serious tissue loss.

Clark goes on to explain the consequences:

The damage done by reactive oxygen molecules needed to operate living cells can be enormous. No molecular species is immune. Oxygen radicals can attack and deform protein molecules, disrupting structural complexes and inhibiting important enzymatic functions. Protein degradation products frequently show up in the body fluids of elderly persons or of patients with chronic infections or chronic inflammatory diseases such as arthritis. Various lipid oxidation products show up in pigment granules called lipofuscin that clog the cells of older individuals, and are a major component of atherosclerotic plaques. Oxygen radicals also attack the individual nucleotide bases that make up both nuclear and mitochondrial DNA.

It is clear that a chronic infection, because it activates the immune system, can cause destruction of cell membranes, organs, and other tissue and even DNA. We have made observations of the immune system cells using the ALCAT test and have seen that nearly everyone exhibits a reaction of the innate immune system initiated by exposure to common foods, additives, and other substances, identical to the reaction just described by William Clark. The inference is that the foods and other substances we are exposed to every day, if incompatible with our own unique biochemical makeup, will result in immune system creation of free radicals and cause the type of physical damage and premature aging Clark describes.

Another immune system glitch involves atherosclerosis. Ever since a Russian physiologist named Nikolai Anitschow reported in the early 20th century that he could induce the disease in rabbits by feeding them a diet high in fats and cholesterol, it has been widely accepted that a diet high in fats and cholesterol is responsible for this disease. Anitschow observed the formation of fatty streaks within the arterial walls of his test animals.

However, in the late 1970s Dr. S. Peng and Dr. K. T. Lee, from Harvard Medical School, using the same species of rabbits, found that a diet high in purified cholesterol (99.99% pure cholesterol) did not reproduce the disease. The explanation for this discrepancy can be found in the work of a German researcher in the late 19th century, named Rudolf Virchow. Dr. Virchow performed numerous autopsies on subjects who had died from heart disease and observed that these patients' arteries appeared as though they had been wounded, suggesting an inflammatory process mediated by the immune system. In light of modern knowledge this observation makes sense.

Today we know that it is not the pure cholesterol that initiates the arterial plaque formation that underlies hardening of the arteries. Instead, it is cholesterol oxides, that is, cholesterol damaged by free radicals, caused by activation of the immune system, which initiates this disease process. The causes? Certainly deficiencies in our antioxidant defense systems play a role, but more than that, anything that causes chronic activation of the innate immune system is the ultimate cause. This, of course, includes immune activation induced by food and environmental sensitivities.

Two Main Branches
of the Immune System

As already discussed, there are two main branches of the immune system—the innate immune system and the adaptive immune system. The distinction between them is a bit theoretical because they interact with each other so intimately. The innate immune system is the branch that is most associated with delayed-onset symptoms of food and chemical intolerance, which is what the ALCAT test deals with. The adaptive, or specific, immune system, is more closely associated with "true allergy," where symptom onset is rapid, more dramatic and acute, and where the association with the ingested food, or chemical, is obvious; thus laboratory testing is usually not required in order to make a diagnosis.

The term *allergy* was coined in 1906 by an Austrian physician named von Pirquet. It meant "altered reaction." Thus any pathological response to a normally benign substance was referred to as an altered reaction, or allergy. It could be the outcome of either innate or adaptive immunity. However, a few decades later, allergists in Europe decided to narrow this definition to describe only such a reaction as occurs in rapid response to exposure to an allergen, such as the appearance of hives immediately following ingestion of shellfish, or a sudden burst of sneezing following the inhalation of dust.

The operative word here is "rapid." When such a reaction concerns a food, the very nature of the reaction, being immediate or very near immediate, makes identifying the specific culprit food quite easy, and there is little need of testing. These are functions of the adaptive or *specific* immune system.

This contrasts with the body's reaction to delayed or hidden food allergies, usually referred to as sensitivities or intolerances, in which symptom onset may take several hours to a couple of days to occur. Hence, delayed food allergies are much more difficult to diagnose, which is why they are called "hidden." It is these types of reactions that the ALCAT test addresses.

When a classic allergy reaction to a food occurs, as a function of the adaptive immune system, identification is easy because the symptoms occur immediately after ingestion. However, immediate, or "classic," allergy reactions to airborne substances may be difficult to identify, because the air contains so many different things at any given time. Thus diagnostic testing, using either skin response or blood testing, is appropriate for airborne allergens. These techniques, however, don't work for delayed reactions to foods, chemicals, and other substances, which arise primarily from activation of the innate immune system.

It is easy to see that knowing what foreign substances and common foods activate the innate immune system is of great importance. Unlike classic allergy symptoms, which are relatively easy to pinpoint, with today's technology, making that identification accurately for delayed food reactions has not been so easy. But that is what the ALCAT test is all about.

Testing for Airborne Allergies

Airborne allergies are fairly easy to diagnose because they are a function of the specific immune system. Use of the word *specific* here means that the immune system is reacting to a specific item. It is also called adaptive immunity, because the immune system reaction adapts to react against the specific item. The process is a little complicated, but it's well understood.

A brief history of the testing for both classic and hidden allergies is useful to understand why the latter type has not received the recognition it is due. For decades, what caused the so-called classic or immediate allergy reactions was not known; however, allergists referred to the unknown agent as reagin. In 1967, two independent teams of researchers, one from the Karolinska Institute in Sweden, and a husband-and-wife team in Colorado named Ishizaka, identified reagin as an IgE antibody. "Ig" in medical speak means "immunoglobulin." Immunoglobulin E (IgE) is the least common of the five major antibody types produced by the immune system.

Through further investigation, these researchers discovered how IgE (now understood to be the reaginic antibody) happens to cause the familiar symptoms of classic allergy—namely, increased mucus secretion and blood vessel permeability; smooth muscle constriction, inflammation, dilation of blood vessels, and stimulation of nerve endings; itching, general discomfort, and pain.

When a foreign protein enters the body, either through inhalation, direct contact with the skin, or ingestion, it may or may not make it through the initial defenses set up at the point of entry. If the foreign substance does get past the barricade, a cell, such as a macrophage (meaning "big eater") or dendritic cell, may absorb it. The cell's internal machinery then breaks down the protein and transports the broken-down peptides on to the cell's own surface. The macrophage or other cell performing this function, such as a dendritic cell, is called an antigen-presenting cell.

In the blood, lymph, and certain specialized tissue exist certain types of white blood cells known as lymphocytes. Different types of lymphocytes do different things. A

T-helper II lymphocyte, or T-cell for short, responds to the presentation of an allergen or antigen (*antigen* means antibody generator). "T-cells" get their name because they mature in the thymus, whereas B-lymphocytes or "B-cells" are so named because they mature in the bone marrow. The T-cell initiates the response. To do so it must "recognize" the specific antigen; that is, it must have a receptor on its surface that conforms to the shape of the peptides of the allergen that is being presented.

If it does conform—and this is the basis of specific immunity—that T-cell and only those T-cells with the same receptor type, is switched on and becomes activated. The activated T-cell then binds with another type of lymphocyte known as a B-lymphocyte if, and only if, the B-cell also shares the same molecular structure, or receptor, on its surface. Thus we see that the immune system has come to recognize and react against a specific allergen. That is why this function is called specific immunity.

In the next step a chemical signal is then transmitted from the T-cell to the B-cell. The B-cell gets switched on, transforms itself into a plasma cell, and begins to manufacture and then secrete soluble forms of that very same type of receptor into the blood. This soluble form of the receptor is an antibody, or immunoglobulin (globule of immunity). Remember, this type of receptor, or antibody, has a shape on one part of it that complements the original shape of the allergen components that started this whole sequence of events. Therefore, it tends to bind with that allergen whenever the two come within close proximity to one another. This is an important point.

As mentioned, those soluble receptors are called antibodies. If the intercellular signal sent from the T-cell to the B-cell involves a chemical called IL4, or interleukin 4, the antibody that the B-cell secretes is of the IgE type. The IgE antibody, like other antibodies, has a "Y" shape to it. The stem portion of the "Y" has the propensity to bind with receptors on yet another type of white blood cell, a mast cell, or a similar type of cell known as a basophil. Mast cells are located in tissues, such as the mucosal lining of the gastrointestinal tract, the respiratory tract, the genitourinary tract, and the skin. Basophils, like mast cells, contain histamine, but they circulate in the blood.

Once bound to the mast cell or basophil, the portion of the IgE antibodies that remains unbound is the part that expresses the molecular configuration complementary to the shape of the peptides of the original allergen. Thus, it is known as an allergen-specific antibody. The next time that allergen comes around, it binds to the exposed portions of the allergen-specific IgE antibodies. When this happens, the mast cell or basophil reacts and the cell membrane breaks down. This allows the small granules within the cells, which contain histamine, to be spewed out and cause the various allergy symptoms. The process, known as degranulation, happens quite quickly.

The immune system is believed to have evolved this particular response to defend against parasites, relatively large entities as compared to white blood cells. Therefore to effectively deter parasites this dramatic spewing of poisonous chemicals is necessary. Why it occurs under inappropriate circumstances, such as a response to ragweed pollen, for instance, is unknown; but the tendency is inherited. On the positive side, people who tend to express this type of allergy, known as atopy, are in fact less susceptible to parasitic infections.

Following the initial distress caused by the release of preformed mediators (such as histamine, in this case), the immune system later converts the phospholipids, which make up the membranes of the involved cells, into other inflammatory mediator types. These mediators, known as lipid mediators and including prostaglandins and leukotrienes, are responsible for the so-called late-phase reaction, which takes place some six to eight hours later and lasts much longer than the initial reaction. Some leukotrienes can constrict the smooth muscles of the bronchial tube 30 times more effectively than histamine.

In his 1997 book *The Zone,* Dr. Barry Sears points out that these mediators are actually autocrine hormones, and can also have an effect on metabolism. Some of them inhibit the burning of fat and/or, induce the storage of fat.

Because the pathway of classic allergy is so well understood it is relatively easy to test for. The first of the two approaches most commonly used is a skin test, which brings the allergen into direct contact with the mast cells in the skin. If the mast cells are coated with IgE antibodies that are specific to the test allergen, a classic reaction involving histamine release, swelling, and redness will occur. This is a time-tested method and a favorite of conventional allergists.

The second approach involves a cleverly devised laboratory test which actually quantifies the levels of allergen-specific IgE antibodies in the blood serum. This more modern approach is more convenient, rapid, and considerably less uncomfortable. And because IgE antibodies are almost always involved in classic allergy reactions, it is nearly as accurate as skin testing.

Testing for Hidden Food Allergies
or Intolerances

With adverse delayed reactions to foods, the diagnosis is much more difficult. IgE antibodies are not involved. Nor is the reaction limited to just the mast cells. In fact, it appears that all the subtypes of immune system cells, especially the phagocytic cells, are involved in these reactions, and these cells are not in the skin. Thus skin tests and antibody tests are not accurate. What is needed to make an accurate identification of an offending food or substance is either a lengthy elimination and challenge procedure, carried out over a period of months, reintroducing one food at a time, no more frequently than one every three days; or a blood test that can measure the reaction of all the immune system cells regardless of what factor or factors that may trigger the reaction. That is why we developed the ALCAT test.

The ALCAT test is aimed at identifying delayed or hidden food allergies, often referred to as sensitivities, intolerances, or simply, adverse reactions. It also tests for other food items, drug and environmental substances. The reactions occur as a result of various biological pathways. Whereas the pathway, or mechanism, underlying classic allergy (where symptom onset is immediate) is very well known, the mechanisms underlying delayed reactions are different and various. Most likely, they are the immune system cells reacting to a chemical that either naturally occurs in a food or is added to it at some stage.

The reaction may also be against complexes of chemicals or natural food constituents, comprised of both proteins and carbohydrates, known as lectins. Dr. Peter D'Adamo has pointed out research going back to the beginning of the 20th century when Dr. Karl Landsteiner first identified inherited differences of "blood type" based on red blood cell surface antigens. Three types were identified: A, B, and O. (Type O blood does not have any of these class of antigens on the red blood cell surface and therefore, Type O people are considered universal donors.) Later Type AB was identified.

Not only was this factor critical when considering blood donations, but some investigators in the 1920s also found associations between particular blood types and specific diseases. For instance, relationships were seen between Types A and B and higher incidences of both alcoholism and heart disease. In 1993, in the British medical journal *The Lancet*, Dr. H. O. Hein and colleagues at the University of Copenhagen Medical School also reported a greater risk of diabetes for these types. Type O people are more prone to gastrointestinal disorders.

Susceptibility to different micro-organisms is also seen among the different blood types, and there is no doubt, that to the extent that a lectin produces an adverse reaction to the associated food, blood type does have some predictive value. However, there are many factors within a food and any one of them may be responsible for activating the immune system. We also have other unique characteristics apart from blood type that determine our sensitivities. Therefore the blood-typing system, although it may give general information in predicting reactions to a food, is too nonspecific to be of adequate help to most people trying to structure an optimal individualized eating plan. However, further research of the relation of blood types to food sensitivities and other predispositions may yield valuable information.

In analyzing the causes of food intolerance, we see that when food passes through the intestinal wall it then enters the portal circulation, which then passes through the liver. Toxic components are modified in the liver during a two-phase process; transformation and then conjugation with other molecules that allow them to be eliminated from the body. Those toxins that go through the first phase are called toxic intermediates, and they can be more damaging to the body than the original toxin. If the second phase of conjugation cannot keep up with the first phase, then some of these toxic intermediates enter the general circulation. Here the immune system cells take a crack at them, and this produces the effects mediated by free radicals, described earlier.

Three major factors contribute to this process:

1. **A hyperpermeable gut (*leaky gut syndrome*),** which can be caused by a number of factors, including irritation, an

imbalance in the types of micro-organisms in the gut
(possibly induced by antibiotic use) an underlying allergic condition directly affecting the gut, and a deficiency
in a certain type of protective antibody complex, called
secretory IgA. When the immune system gets cranked
up, the adrenal glands will produce more cortisol. Excess cortisol can cause both gut hyperpermeability and
a deficiency in secretory IgA antibodies. Thus stress,
which raises cortisol levels, can also contribute to food
sensitivities in this way. Stress also weakens the immune
system in other ways. Whatever the cause, incompletely
digested food particles are more likely to activate the
immune system than are fully digested food particles.

2. **A slow or deficient detoxification pathway** fails to eliminate toxins, which are then dealt with by the immune
system cells. In some instances a particular detoxification pathway may be overwhelmed because there is too
much toxin to handle. This can occur because a certain
detoxification enzyme is deficient. Just as a deficiency in
a digestive enzyme makes it difficult or impossible to digest a certain food substance, as when lactase deficiency
inhibits digestion of lactose (milk sugar), a detoxification enzyme deficiency makes it difficult or impossible
to break down a dietary toxin. Many detox enzymes also
require cofactors: micronutrients, such as vitamins and
minerals, which should be in the diet. However, commercial agricultural practices deplete the soil of its natural mineral content. If it's not in the soil, then it's not
in the diet.

Thus the modern diet consisting primarily of processed and adulterated foods contributes to food sensitivities in two ways: It introduces more unnatural and
foreign substances into the body, and it does not provide adequate levels of nutrients necessary for proper
liver detoxification. Sometimes a large dose of a foreign

chemical so overwhelms a detox pathway that the body then develops a sensitivity to new foods or chemicals that contain chemically related components. The initial insult that sets up the sensitivity is called induction. The body's subsequent reactivity to chemically related substances is called spreading.

3. **A genetic predisposition to react to a particular food substance.** Some genetic tendencies are associated with place of origin. For example, compared to Caucasians most Japanese do not have as much alcohol dehydrogenase, the enzyme that breaks down the ethyl alcohol in alcoholic beverages. Thus a businessman of Japanese genetic heritage may get drunk more quickly and remain intoxicated longer than his Caucasian-heritage counterpart of the same size and weight, drinking the same amount of alcohol. In Japan, the business culture has adapted to this phenomenon, and it is even encouraged that Japanese co-workers regularly have social drinks together, as it is during these moments of intoxication that the workers can express normally repressed sentiments about work-related issues. In this way discussions of this nature can take place that are not acceptable within the context of the rather austere business setting during daytime periods of sobriety. This inherited tendency thus serves a useful social and business purpose.

Similarly, most of the world population is lactose intolerant after childhood. Thus Americans of African and Asian heritage are also more likely to produce less lactase than do those of northern European (Caucasian) descent. In January 2002, Dr. Leena Peltonen, a geneticist from UCLA, and her team isolated the gene that causes lactose intolerance, which affects between 30 and 50 million Americans, most of them of African and Asian descent. Only about 5 percent of descendents of northern Europeans do not produce lactase, the enzyme that breaks down lactose. Of course, babies of all peoples can digest breast milk, which naturally contains the lactase (contained in mothers' milk). As children from Africa and Asia, as well as Native Americans, get older, they then lose the ability.

Why did some people develop this genetic mutation that allows them to consume dairy product, whereas others did not? Dr. Peltonen says, "We believe that the variant we identified in patients is the original form of the gene—which mutated to tolerate milk products when early humans adopted dairy farming. In cold climates where winter crops cannot be reaped, a gene mutation allowing adults to digest milk would help people survive better. People who survive pass on these genes to their offspring. Ten to twelve thousand years ago, when human populations started to use dairy culture—cattle, goats—around that time the mutation happened and made some individuals lactose tolerant."

Here we see an illustration of how our genetic ancestry, based on thousands of generations of previous exposures, determines our capability to digest a food. No doubt this goes a long way toward explaining today's increased cases of food intolerance. Since commercialized agriculture and food processing began, which was only around 50 or 60 years ago, the food that we eat has now come to resemble less and less the food our ancestors ate. We must take into account factors of human migration, food migration (through preservation and shipping), food adulteration, now modification through genetic manipulation, and less natural nutritional support for the detoxification pathways. And we must also take into account that scientists now believe that chronic activation of the innate immune system underlies diabetes, cardiovascular disease, and obesity. So is it any wonder that such diseases have now reached epidemic proportions in industrialized societies?

New Methods for Testing
Genetic Susceptibilities to Foods?

Just as a tendency to have or not have a digestive or detoxification enzyme may be inherited, so too may a predisposition to react to particular foreign substances. It is well known that food and nutrients affect genetic expression. Every somatic cell in the body contains the entire genome or blueprint for the entire body in its nuclear DNA. A liver cell differs from a skin cell, which differs from a nerve cell, and so on, because each cell only expresses that portion of the person's genome that is involved in the production and function of that particular cell type. Not only are different genes selectively either expressed or left dormant in order for cell differentiation to occur during fetal development, but also, throughout the entire life of the organism, genetic expression within each cell determines cell, tissue, and organ function. The foods we eat and the chemicals we are exposed to, play a major role in how the genes are expressed.

For DNA to express itself appropriately, it relays on the information passed to it through numerous chemical messages originating from many other different cells. How the genes express themselves is very much related to the foods we eat, the chemicals we are exposed to, as well as other lifestyle factors, such as exercise.

In 1993 researcher Dr. C. Ezzell reported in *Science News,* in a paper entitled "Awakened Gene Aids Inherited Anemias," that two nutrient substances, butyrate and hydroxyuria, are capable of "awakening" that portion of the DNA that encodes for the proteins that make up the fetal hemoglobin molecule in adults suffering from sickle cell anemia. Sickle cell anemia is a genetic disease characterized by a defect in the formation of the adult hemoglobin molecule on red blood cells, which carries oxygen. When the fetal hemoglobin gene is awakened in this manner, it overrides the defective genetic message and "dilutes" the misformed hemoglobin molecule, thus improving the condition. Here we see an example of a nutritional intervention positively affecting genetic espression in order to treat a specific medical condition. However, note that in its region of origin, Africa, the sickle cell trait, when not fully expressed, helps protect against malaria, which is endemic there.

The modern diet consisting primarily of processed and adulterated foods contributes to food sensitivities in two ways: It introduces more unnatural and foreign substances into the body, and it does not provide adequate levels of nutrients necessary for proper liver detoxification.

Scientists have recently developed new tools to rapidly determine which genes are expressed in response to stimuli in the environment of the cell. They are called microarrays, and they consist of microscopic bits of DNA bound onto little pieces of glass. When DNA becomes expressed, it creates a mirror image template of its unique chemical structure out of messenger RNA (mRNA), which then migrates to another part of the cell, the ribosomes, where the associated protein is assembled. Pieces of messenger RNA tagged with fluorescent labels are then exposed to the hundreds of DNA sequences bound on the glass. When the matching mRNA and DNA bind, they emit a measurable glow that indicates the activation of the DNA in the cell from which the sample came.

By using this method scientists can determine how changing the environment, or the nutrients the cell receives, causes different genes to be expressed. Dr. R. K. Blanchard and his team at Food Science and Human Nutrition Department and Center for Nutritional Sciences, at the University of Florida at Gainsville, reported (in November 2001 in the *Proceedings of the National Academy of Science*) how a zinc deficiency negatively affects the expression of genes that control several important physiological processes, including energy use. They believe that their approach may someday be used to determine individual nutritional status.

The ALCAT test provides a much simpler approach to determining which foods and substances induce the expression of genes that promote health. Regardless of the pathway, or biological mechanism, the immune system cells "know" when a food or substance may harm the body. Unlike specific or adaptive immunity, in which there must be an initial exposure to establish recognition and in which reaction only occurs following repeated or prolonged exposure, many of the delayed type of adverse reactions are actually programmed into the genes.

For example, we have observed that children who have been raised on a kosher diet (which allows no pork) will show a reaction to pork on the first exposure of pork to the blood cells through the ALCAT test. This phenomenon is reminiscent of the tradition of Indians in the U.S. Southwest, who are advised to avoid close contact with rodents that carry the hanta virus; these animals are deadly to them but not to other racial groups. Thus there appears to be biological wisdom in the religion-based health dicta of certain ethnic groups (orthodox Jews and Muslims do not eat pork; orthodox Hindus do not eat beef; and so forth).

There is no way to predetermine what strategy the immune system may implement to counter the effects of a foreign substance. To identify the offending substance, it is necessary to implement a measurement that is a final common pathway of all mechanisms. Such a pathway is represented by the total population of the immune system cells, or leukocytes.

The ALCAT test looks at the changes in both the size and the number of the leukocytes after the whole blood has been exposed to the battery of test substances, usually consisting of 100 to 153 food items plus food additives, colorings, environmental chemicals, and sometimes other individual potential "allergens" according to the patient's needs. The method of measuring the cells uses an electronic instrument that is capable of discerning these changes with great sensitivity. The method is referred to as the impedance or "Coulter" method, after the late Wallace Coulter, who invented it. It has been used routinely for many years in hematologic laboratory analysis (the study of blood).

The story of the invention is quite interesting. When Coulter was a young man, he had a job counting fish. One day he had the clever idea of narrowing the channel through which the fish swam such that only one fish could swim through at a time. He then rigged an electrical device that would generate an electrical current across the channel capable of detecting a drop in electrical voltage should it occur. The body of a fish will not conduct electricity as well as water and therefore impedes the electrical current. Later, he sophisticated the concept and adapted it to a microscopic level for use in measuring microscopic particles, such as blood cells (see Figure 4.1).

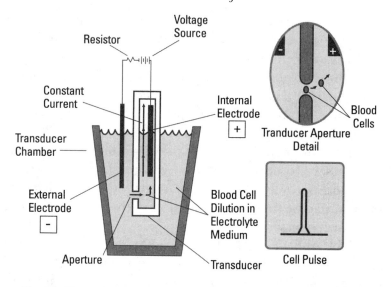

Fig. 4.1. The methodology used by the ALCAT test to measure blood cells.

The ALCAT test measurements are performed on the whole blood within 28 hours of blood draw. During this time all the elements that may be involved in an adverse reaction—including all the blood cells, antibodies, serum proteins, and cytokines (chemical messengers produced at the cellular level)—are still alive and viable. In this way, the test mimics, as closely as possible, what actually happens when food products and other foreign substances reach the blood.

This method of testing is in some respects analogous to skin testing, where the allergen is placed into contact with the histamine containing cells in the skin. However, it is much more sophisticated, because the "allergen" is placed directly into contact with the whole live blood, where it is able to interact with all the immune system cells as well as other factors (see Figure 4.2). Therefore it can show a reaction regardless of what biological pathway

Sample Reaction Histograms

Master Control   Test Sample

Fig. 4.2. When the presence of an allergen in the blood causes a reaction, it is easily seen because it causes a change in either the size and/or number of white cells or activation of platelets.

causes it. The method of measurement is also electronic, so it is objective and reproducible. This is why it has such a high level of correlation with clinical symptoms, meaning that it is highly accurate.

Well-controlled studies have shown a high degree of correlation with double-blind oral challenges with foods and food additives. Use of the test then provides accurate and valuable information that could only otherwise be obtained through a lengthy elimination-and-challenge procedure. It is the only blood test for this purpose that has this characteristic.

Individual Biochemistry:
No "One Size Fits All" Diet

Just as no single mechanism lies behind all food intolerance, no two people with food intolerance are the same. For one thing, an aspect of genetics, called genetic polymorphism, affects all types of reactions that might be associated with symptoms caused by food. Genetic polymorphism is what makes each of us different, despite the fact that our genetic makeup is almost identical. This means that distinct types of factors are uniquely common to a group of people within the human species—for example, Mediterraneans or Eskimos. These groups have different enzymes or enzymes that operate at a unique rate. If your ancestors were never exposed to a particular food, it's likely you and others in your group never developed a genetic predisposition to deal with it enzymatically. Thus different groups react to food, its metabolism, and its toxicity in different ways.

What's more, within these groups each individual's biochemistry is completely unique. Although primarily inherited, it is also affected by environment, lifestyle, health, and other experiences. As such, each person with food intolerance has different symptoms, which vary in degree, age of onset, duration, location, and amount of food needed to trigger the symptoms. The same food can produce vastly different symptoms in different people, and different foods can cause different symptoms in the same person. So, before you have eaten even one mouthful of food, several scenarios are possible. These factors explain why no one single diet can fit every person's nutritional and health needs. Only an individualized diet, which eliminates your intolerant foods, can help ensure that allergens and toxins that interfere with maximum health do not overload your system.

*Only an individualized diet, which
eliminates your intolerant foods, can
help ensure that allergens and toxins
that interfere with maximum health
do not overload your system.*

When we are sick, something in the body is wrong. It's clear from this brief explanation the multitude of problems that can occur in our digestive system, immune system, and enzymatic system. Doctors who practice preventive medicine agree that when any one of these systems is not working, a person has taken a step further away from optimal health. The goal of maximum health is to get these processes and others working at optimum performance. Once you get these systems healthy, you've taken a giant step to enabling your body to use these dynamic and powerful systems to take care of itself. Clearly, if you remove food to which you are intolerant, you'll give your body a fighting chance to clear up the migraines, joint pains, fatigue, skin problems, excess weight, and other health problems triggered and compounded by foods. Identifying and removing reactive foods is the key to your good health.

CHAPTER 5

Overweight: As American As Apple Pie

If you are reading this book we both know one thing; whatever you are eating isn't working.

Contemporary medicine seeks to satisfy the needs and demands of an ever-growing population of overweight Americans by prescribing drugs that work on appetite suppression, serotonin levels, and the binding of fat in the intestine. Although many studies suggest these treatments work, we still treat obesity blindly. Few patients are getting well, and we don't know why people are getting more and more overweight.

The following statement from the *Journal of the American Medical Association* (*JAMA*, vol. 272, issue 3, July 20, 1994) summarizes the results of four separate large national studies pertaining to obesity:

> Understanding the underlying reasons for the increased prevalence of overweight in the United States and elucidating the potential consequences for health outcomes challenge our understanding of the etiology, treatment, and

prevention of overweight. Overweight is increasing in U.S. adults and continues to be a public health dilemma for which no efficacious, practical, and long-lasting preventive or therapeutic solution has yet been identified.

Why Are We Overweight?

At the disposal of every American is the "food pyramid," put forth by the U.S. Department of Agriculture as the appropriate proportions of fats, proteins, and carbohydrates to keep us healthy. Healthy, perhaps—but it certainly won't trim our waistline. Endless studies show that eating too much will cause weight gain, more studies show that taking medication causes weight loss, and even more enlightening studies prove if you change what you do you won't do it any more (lifestyle change). Give me a break! Of all the diseases, obesity would seem obviously caused by an abnormal reaction to food. The clue is that in spite of all the theories, Americans continue to gain weight.

Whether alone or in conjunction, accepted therapies for overweight often don't work for the long term. Their weakness lies in the inaccurate premise that every individual is identical in digestion, metabolism, and function. If this were true, why aren't we all presidents? The fact is that despite all the scientific study and analysis, humans defy general categorization. Each of us differs in the way we respond to food, oxygen, chemicals, and even visual and sensory input. We are as different in our reaction to foods as in our political philosophies.

The documented biochemical progression of food through our bodies does not explain our overweight or abnormal cravings for food. We don't have the full picture; we're overlooking some factor. To date the great majority of research has been directed toward developing medications to treat symptoms of hunger and cravings. Given the incredible amount of money to be made in the field of antiobesity medication—to help people lose the same pound of fat over and over—why would drug companies spend money researching the role of food intolerance? Which among them is going to shoot the goose laying the golden eggs?

Donna Ryan, M.D., stated that "more than one in three Americans are overweight . . . up from one in four Americans a little more than a decade earlier." The most recent statistics now show that nearly two out of three Americans are overweight. In five short years the numbers seem to have almost doubled. We must agree with her conclusion:

> One would think that the emphasis on managed care would spur a reassessment of the need for preventative approaches. Obesity contributes directly and indirectly to chronic disease risk, and measures to ameliorate and prevent the disorder should receive top priority for research funding. ("Medicating the Obese Patient," *Endocrinology and Metabolism Clinics of North America,* vol. 25, issue 4, December 1996)

The relationship of food intolerance to overweight is like the relationship of gasoline to fire: Gasoline may cause the fire and will surely keep it raging. So suggestive is the relationship that I routinely recommend that people with a history of "yo-yo dieting" get tested for food intolerance. Furthermore, if overweight patients have concurrent symptoms associated with food sensitivities, testing is even more imperative. If food intolerance is what has kept them sick or caused the regain of weight, they need to know this before they can hope to keep off the weight. And avoiding foods is much safer than taking medication for the long term.

Why Am I Paying for Insurance?

The numbers may vary among the many studies and polls done to determine the frequency of overweight in America. But the fact is that between 60 percent and 80 percent of us are at risk for premature death, social stigmatization, and the concurrent medical conditions associated with overweight and obesity. It is mind-boggling that under these circumstances health insurance companies are allowed to exclude treatment of overweight as a cosmetic condition. Allowing the insurance companies to continue to deny treatment is akin to allowing people to die lying at the bottom of a hole because the hole they have fallen into isn't deep enough by some bureaucratic definition. Any other insurance is held to a different standard from that of health insurance. If you buy roadside assistance insurance, you get help when you need it regardless of whether bad judgment led to your distress or not. Your auto insurance carrier can't refuse to pay because you used poor judgment and became involved in an accident. Certainly such insurance carriers can promptly charge you a higher premium after you have proven to be a higher risk, but it is nonetheless their duty to live up to the promise they made you. Can you imagine an insurance company refusing to repair body damage after an accident because the damage was only cosmetic? We take better care of our cars than we do our bodies.

The North American Association for the Study of Obesity is the nation's leading scientific society dedicated to the study of obesity. In a news release in March 2002, Dr. Charles Billington, M.D. (immediate past president of NAASO, member of the National Task Force on the Prevention and Treatment of Obesity, and professor of medicine at the University of Minnesota in Minneapolis) concluded, "We must begin to view obesity as a medical problem and reimburse for appropriate treatments. It seems illogical that insurance payers are willing to pay for the treatment of diseases such as diabetes, abnormal blood lipids, hypertension, and heart disease, but will not pay for the treatment of obesity, which is often the underlying cause of these diseases." NAASO has been actively working with the Surgeon General, Congress, the U.S. Department of Agriculture (USDA), and the National Institutes of Health (NIH) to address obesity and recognizes reimbursement as a key issue in reversing the epidemic.

Dr. Billington added, "Providing treatment for obesity will lead to improved health for millions of Americans. NAASO urges increased accessibility for treatment. The epidemic can be reversed with the right support." It bears repeating at this juncture that obesity resulted in the loss of 300,000 lives and a cost of $117 billion in the year 2000 alone. We are off to a dismal start to the 21st century.

Health insurance reimbursement must be made accessible for those suffering from overweight and obesity, and it must be paid for. Just as it would be unconscionable to allow people who had fallen into a pit to die without trying to help get them out, it is a national disgrace for us to abandon those dying in the epidemic of obesity. What is the sense in spending billions of dollars stockpiling antibiotics and vaccines to maybe protect some of us from some possible future terrorist threat and not address a preventable condition that is consistently killing 300,000 of us every year and costing us $117 billion dollars a year in medical costs? It seems that the perception of overweight people as second-rate deeply permeates our culture. Forget race, gender, and religious discrimination; we are talking about a statistically confirmed health epidemic that crosses all those categories that is being not so elegantly dodged, sidestepped, and denied. It just doesn't carry the media appeal, political popularity, or shock value of a mysterious white powder that may be delivered through the mail.

As a nation in denial, we must come to our senses. We must address this epidemic head on and rescue the 300,000 Americans at the bottom of the pit this year while at the same time throw a rope to the millions of others willing to climb out on their own with just a little help. Those suffering needlessly from overweight for lack of finances or guidance flounder hopelessly in the "land of plenty." If the statistics are correct, and I have no doubt they are, the 60 percent to 80 percent of Americans who are overweight have the political wherewithal to insist that they receive the medical attention they deserve. And when this massive block of voters decides to change the system for the better, we will become a more reality-based democracy. Message to the powers that be: "Come home, we have big problems here. We are being ignored, humiliated, killed and economically ravaged by the very system you created and we sustain."

While we all wait for someone else to take the time and make the sacrifices to change a slow-to-change system, we must take matters of our health to heart. For those able to help themselves, there is opportunity. We must stop contracting out our health care and must take full control individually. Most of the things we go to a doctor for are a result of something we should have eaten and didn't, or shouldn't have eaten and did. You do not have to go to medical school to take care of your human body. It came with preprogrammed instructions, you just aren't following them. Turn the TV off, go for a long walk, then come home and start reading about healthy eating, avoiding overweight, and how to care for your children through their diet. Look into food sensitivity testing, learn the foods your body runs best on, and eat them. It is all on the line every day, and in the battle for your health if you aren't winning, you are losing.

The Serotonin Made Me Do It

Finally a logical explanation for the heretofore uncontrollable desire to eat inappropriate foods at inappropriate times has surfaced: You crave chocolate tonight because of your allergic response to the carrots you ate yesterday. Simply put, the allergic reaction depleted serotonin in your system. Responding to your brain's flashing red warning lights of low serotonin, you subconsciously search out foods to increase brain serotonin levels.

"Wait a minute!" the enlightened among you may cry, "How can eating a piece of bread, mostly carbohydrate, cause an increase in a protein hormone in the brain?" This may be the time to clarify how serotonin fits into this picture. Serotonin is produced in the brain. It cannot get into the brain from the bloodstream. To produce serotonin, the brain must have precursors in the form of certain amino acid building blocks.

Amino acids are the smallest building blocks that the body uses to make proteins it needs as hormones. The specific precursor to serotonin is tryptophan, an amino acid. Tryptophan is special in that it is pretty scarce in the bloodstream. Most other amino acids are branched-chain amino acids and are fairly plentiful compared to tryptophan.

At any rate, all these amino acids line up at the blood-brain barrier waiting their turn to be transported to the brain. The blood-brain barrier is like the border between countries. The body is very particular as to what gets through the blood-brain barrier, and a backup develops. Meanwhile the level of serotonin in the brain continues to fall. Your brain tells you to go eat something sweet. As soon as you do that, your insulin level soars.

The immediate effect of insulin in the bloodstream is to direct all the branched-chain amino acids to their respective posts to begin building muscle hormones and enzymes to take advantage of the sugary energy you have just eaten. The insulin sweeps through all the amino acids in line at the blood-brain barrier, conscripting all those that are branched-chain amino acids for duties elsewhere in the body. Tryptophan, normally not one of the more common amino acids, now finds itself highly concentrated at the blood-brain barrier, by the insulin tidal wave.

Subsequently more tryptophan enters the brain more quickly and is promptly converted to serotonin, one of the neurotransmitters responsible for determining hunger. As serotonin levels rise, the need to feed disappears and the body assumes a well-fed, calm, peaceful state. As serotonin levels decay, this process repeats itself. The whole process is thrown into action each and every time serotonin levels drop below a certain set point for that individual. External factors may also deplete serotonin. These include long-term stress, sleep deprivation, illness, and food sensitivity reactions. Regardless of the precipitating event, the bodily urge to raise serotonin levels manifests as a strong craving for a food that will raise insulin levels and replenish serotonin levels rapidly. This is why you crave sweets.

A survey conducted in 2002 by the Chocolate Manufacturers Association was released in conjunction with the celebration of "American Chocolate Week, March 17–23." I had to smile as I read the results of the poll of 1,022 U.S. women surveyed. Some of the strongly supportive views quoted (remember, this study was conducted by a group who wants you to eat more chocolate) include the following:

> In addition to pure enjoyment, 52 percent of women said eating chocolate makes them happy.
>
> Forty-six percent of women noted that they eat chocolate as a pick-me-up.
>
> Thirty-five percent said eating chocolate simply makes them feel good.

Sixty-five percent of women surveyed said they eat
chocolate candy or chocolate desserts at least weekly,
while 15 percent said they enjoy chocolate daily.

These women were self-medicating. They were using
food for its psychoactive drug effects: to improve mood, boost
energy, and provide a general sense of well being. Not so curiously, absent in the survey is the incidence of overweight, diabetes, heart disease, and high cholesterol in the study
group. In this case a small, skewed survey is designed to support those readers looking for some validation for their own
cravings. I have no particular antagonism toward chocolate,
or better said, toward the cocoa bean, which, in fact, contains
antioxidants. I do have some serious reservations about the
health value of chocolate-flavored sugar. But for a group who
is profiting from a product to present their own study, which
simply states that these women feel a certain way about their
product, in no way commits the group. I can't help but wonder if a study of cocaine addicts might not get similar support
from the study participants. I wonder why there isn't a "Stop
Eating Sugar Week"? Maybe they just ran out of weeks that
could be named before they ran out of candies.

Down Insulin! Down! Bad Insulin!

One chemical reaction in the body leads to another in perpetual motion. Serotonin aside, we now have raging insulin
levels as the body tries to take advantage of the precious
sugar energy you have consumed. Insulin will direct the
blood glucose (sugar) into the muscle cells and liver, where
it can be stored for future use as glycogen. You are unlikely
to need it immediately because of your current drowsy state
resulting from elevated serotonin levels. Not one to waste
energy resources once all the storage capacity for glycogen

is filled, the body directs the conversion of excess glucose into fat. And it doesn't take too long before that storage capacity in the muscle tissue and liver is reached.

Once this occurs, the effect of insulin is to open the fat cell to accept fat for storage and close off the release of fat from the cell into the bloodstream. This is because the body preferentially uses glucose as an energy source over fat, when it is available. This is a good example of what is called a cascade. That is, a sugary food (or food having a high glycemic index) is consumed, insulin is produced, the sugars are stored in fat cells as fat and not burned for energy requirements, lack of energy is felt, then more sugar is consumed.

If you are someone who exercises regularly, eats "right," and still can't lose weight, think about the possibility that you may have food sensitivities.

The end result is that you are lethargic, with a full tank of energy stored as both glycogen and fat. Because your serotonin level is fine, your only tendency to eat is from a fluctuating insulin level, causing you to seek sweets to correct your hypoglycemia.

This is a nightmare of perpetual bad news for the overweight patient. Elevated serotonin levels and intermittent hypoglycemia keep one lethargic, while increased insulin levels promote storing more energy as fat. You can tell right now, the scales are not going to be kind tomorrow!

Yes, food sensitivities can keep you fat. If you are someone who exercises regularly, eats "right," and still can't lose weight, think about the possibility that you may have food sensitivities. You may try to avoid sugary sweets, but probably liberally indulge in pasta, bread, or starches. The body is responding to the lowered serotonin levels resulting from a delayed food sensitivity. These refined grain products may in some cases raise insulin levels as fast or faster than sugar. Compound the dilemma by eating any amount of saturated fat along with your sugar or refined grain treat and stand back: Those fat cells are going to swell. Finding out whether you have a food intolerance that leads you to crave carbohydrates can enable you to put an end to the vicious cycle. Eliminating the foods to which you react badly will result in diminished cravings and a proper resumption of normal metabolic pathways. Weight loss will then follow this normalizing of body functions.

The Agony of "The Feed"

It may sound obvious, but still bears saying: "It's not fun being overweight." I don't know anyone who has said, "Yeah, I think I will totally ignore myself until I weigh 350 pounds." Because this is not one of those noble goals we set for ourselves in high school, it is by default a negative aspect of our adult development. The fact is that the pain and anguish start early as one gains weight. Initially, the pain is one of depriving oneself of food as a pleasure from time to time to control small weight gains. Panic and fear follow this, as short-term dieting no longer does the job. Short-term successes with "quick fix" medication lead to long-term disgust as the pounds come back. Soon denial and guilt obstruct effective treatment. Self-esteem falls off the edge of the table, and depression darkens life. Psychologically, some people may resign themselves to their condition, remaining fat and possibly, especially with teen age girls, desexualizing themselves so as to avoid the emotional pressure of even competing for social acceptance. Those you know who are overweight have or will feel each of these emotions as they slowly withdraw from activities and events they enjoy. Despite their other successes, they live in the shadow of defeat until they get over this final hurdle. Understand their frustration. After all, they were never voted "most likely to be fat."

Doom and Gloom

As we try to lose weight, we unconsciously doom success as we approach each weight loss effort with short-term goals. Perhaps the goals are left from the days when the pounds fell away easily or perhaps stem from denial that we have a serious problem with food. At any rate, we secretly realize that this weight problem is forever. We've read everywhere that more than 90 percent who lose weight gain it back within a year or two. We accept our fate and open our wallets. Desperate to at least give the appearance of making an effort to get the weight off, we proceed from one weight loss gimmick to another. Some actually work for a short period, but the weight always finds its way back. Remember, the multibillion-dollar weight loss industry isn't profitable because it works, it is extremely profitable because it *doesn't*. The same clients are recycled over and over, making each successive unsuccessful program profitable for someone.

Fair-Weather Friends

People close to us seem to flaunt our weakness as they offer food in abundance. Confused as to what would really make us happy, our friends offer the gift we obviously enjoy. Unwilling to bring attention to ourselves, we eat, begrudgingly fitting into the very mold society cast for us. Once started, we now eat to elevate ourselves from the pit of self-pity and guilt with a serotonin surge. We have a disease. No other illness is treated with such callous disregard by society.

We are dying, and no one cares. Others in fact take every opportunity to make money off our misfortune. They tempt us with stories of success and pass us off to the next "90-day wonder" program, knowing we will return. Even many of our doctors don't seem to realize we are sick. We have a ravaging chemical reaction coursing through our bodies and don't know why. Food sensitivities leading to absorptive malnutrition, immune system dysfunction, and multiple organ system symptoms brand us as "chronic disease patients." In the case of allergic reaction to foods, the effect on the body is similar to that of a parasite, which drains the host's reserves of energy, creates imbalances in brain chemistry, and interrupts desirable body functions. To try to keep up nutritionally with this constant drain and waste of body energy would be like trying to fill a tub with water without plugging the drain.

Desperation, psychological defeat, and social ostracism lead us to the dark side of life. Our only hope is that someone will recognize our plight and assist us in identifying the culprit foods.

Encouraged to Eat

Contrary to popular thought, overweight does not result from lack of willpower. Simply pushing away from the table is too easy a concept; it insults the intelligence of patient and doctor. If it were that easy, I assure you there would not be a restaurant on every busy street corner. This drive to eat and overeat is as strong a compulsion as any drug craving, modulated by chemical reactions created in the body by foods. It is big business, capitalized on by big corporations.

Be it the effect on serotonin levels or the stimulation of endorphin receptors, certain people experience a sincere pleasure and euphoria from eating. This sensation is so much preferred over the status quo that we aggressively seek it to avoid the pain of reality. A common behavior in middle-aged patients is a tendency to overeat because they are unhappy with their lives. The pain and disappointment of unfulfilled dreams and expectations is too much to bear. Increased alcohol consumption and its empty calories often precede the history of overeating in these patients. But compared to the undesirable social stigma of excessive alcohol consumption, eating is socially acceptable and even encouraged by society.

Virtually all our social gatherings—from board meetings to celebrating religious festivals—are characterized by abundant food. Maybe this reflects our heritage as humans—to break bread together is a sign of friendship. But the tradition has gotten way out of hand. The overweight individual is placed in the precarious position of either appearing to shun the celebration or becoming an out-of-control eating machine. This no-win proposition leaves most of us choosing to eat ourselves into the euphoria that lets us escape reality. Plainly put, a common cause of overweight is social circumstances that expose those suffering from overweight to the public humiliation of succumbing to addiction. This cruel and irresponsible enticement to food is imposed daily on overweight people.

The Yeast Beast Doth Have Me

Other underlying causes of overweight are more physiological. For example, Jan, a middle-aged woman, came to my office determined to lose weight once and for all. As this was her "many-eth" time, Jan deserves credit for perseverance. In our interview we reviewed the usual eating history and cycle of weight gain and loss she had battled since childhood. Each weight loss had been followed by an equally impressive weight regain. She casually mentioned that she had been a sickly child and had many bouts of throat and ear infections. At one point Jan had been put on a variety of antibiotics for over two months. During her teenage years she put on weight and dealt from that point on with the misery of being overweight. When asked, she told of many bouts with vaginal "yeast" infections, even routinely using vaginal suppositories during her menstrual period in an effort to prevent the relentless infections that followed her cycle. Eventually marriage and pregnancy led to a C-section, followed again by a long course of antibiotics to deal with complications.

The overwhelming evidence revealed that Jan was suffering from candidiasis, an intestinal yeast infestation that can spread systemically. The most common cause of candidiasis is the *candidia albicans* species. It normally grows in the vaginal and intestinal tract but a healthy immune system, under normal conditions, will keep it in check. Certain factors will increase its growth: antibiotics, stress, and immunosuppressive drugs like cortisone, hormonal drugs, like oral contraceptives; viral infections, and heavy metal toxicity. The candida is a type of yeast and will flourish if fed refined carbohydrates (pastries), fermented drinks (like beer and wine), and artificial food additives.

Once established in the intestines the candida releases toxins and potential allergens. It also increases the permeability of the intestines and may damage a certain type of protective immune protein molecule, called secretory IgA, which keeps debris, undigested food particles, and other toxins from entering the blood. When the candida cells die off they release further toxins, creating discomfort. Because the yeast feed off of refined carbohydrates, the infected person will often crave them so as to avoid the unpleasantness associated with the dying candida phenomenon.

Sure enough, when she was specifically asked about sweet and starch cravings, she admitted she craved sweets and especially chocolates in an inhuman way but avoided them for the obvious caloric reasons. She, however, allowed herself to enjoy bread on a daily basis as well as frequent servings of frozen yogurt, baked potatoes, and rice dishes. She had used yogurt at one time to alleviate her monthly yeast infections and associated it with health.

Jan had the ALCAT test done, which confirmed that she had a strong reaction to several foods as well as a reaction to *candida albicans* (yeast). This positive reaction implied that the yeast itself had entered the blood at some time, which made treatment that much more imperative. We had an extended talk about a "candida diet protocol" and her need to avoid all sweets, starches, and "yeast" foods such as bread and alcohol, as well as foods to which she had tested positive on the ALCAT test. An appetite suppressant, phentermine, was prescribed to enable her to stick to the restrictive diet. Jan stayed on her diet, and to make an already long story short, she recovered quite well. Her sweet cravings subsided and, after a month of treatment with an alternative protocol that included caprylic acid, garlic, and oil of oregano for candidiasis, she felt more energetic. Her weight dropped nicely, and she resumed eating responsibly and taking vitamin and mineral supplements to strengthen her immune system. She will be followed routinely to monitor her weight and cravings.

If her sweet cravings flare up again, Jan knows how to use the protocol to treat the yeast, and also knows that she may need to treat it with medication in the future. She understands the value of the rotation diet concept (rotating foods so the same food is not eaten more than once every four days) in preventing food sensitivity and eats a variety of foods. Her advantage is that she now has an option: Jan knows she does not have to be fat, and she has control of her destiny.

Although the connection is not precisely understood, intestinal yeast infections and food intolerance are closely related. Identifying Jan's reactivity to yeast was crucial—offering compelling evidence that aggressive treatment with antifungal medications or alternative protocols while eliminating reactive foods was appropriate. As a matter of fact, for the reasons described above having to do with candida's harmful effects on the intestines and the activation of the immune system, successful treatment of the yeast infection may be necessary to prevent additional food intolerance from developing.

Out with the Good and In with the Bad

With the advent of abundant antibiotics, we may be unaware of the price we pay. Many antibiotics have a devastating effect on the good bacteria in your intestine—bacteria necessary for the complete digestion of food. If these bacteria are eliminated by a prolonged round of antibiotics, the small intestine becomes fertile ground for yeast to colonize. Commonly found in the throat and digestive system of healthy humans, these yeast only become a problem when the immune system is compromised. When not controlled by our immune system, these yeast reproduce rapidly and set up shop in the lining of the intestine. Once established, they can be very hard to eradicate. An estimated 25 million Americans suffer from chronic candidiasis.

Opportunistic Menace

The yeast itself is normally a benign, casual "passerby" in the digestive tract. From the mouth and esophagus to the colon, yeast may be commonly found in healthy people. As with so many infections of the body, everything is okay until it isn't. That is, as long as the body defenses are intact and functioning properly, these casual occupants of the digestive tract are no more threatening than the food digesting therein. However, in the event that the immune system is suppressed, these opportunistic organisms quickly take advantage of the ideal conditions afforded by the intestinal tract. They attach to the lining of the intestine and easily tap into the rich blood supply. Surviving on the sugar and starches, which they ferment to use, they grow and reproduce through spores and through asexual propagation (breaking off of pieces). This dual method of reproduction enables them to propagate in different areas of the intestine by simply breaking apart and reestablishing themselves at a more favorable site.

As the yeast population increases, so do the patient's symptoms. Physical invasion of the intestine lining, along with inflammation associated with the attachment of foreign bodies, prevent the intestinal mucosa from absorbing nutrients as usual. In addition, because the yeast greedily extract nutrients they need for survival, the human host gets less. The immune system cells in the lining of the intestine eventually (remember, it was suppressed) respond and find themselves in a real "David and Goliath" predicament. At the same time, the lining of the intestine, now compromised by this parasite, doesn't function in its usual selective way. Larger-than-normal size particles of food may be absorbed into the bloodstream through the intestinal lining that's inflamed or irritated by the yeast.

This is, in effect, the second alarm turned in to the immune system. It now has to deal with these abnormal "foreign" particles of food as well as continue to attack the yeast. Before long the combination of continuous demand and decreasing nutritional absorption limit the ability of the immune system to function. In an all-out survival war against the yeast and food, the immune system begins to confiscate nutrients from other tissues to carry out its duties. Now fighting the war with a shrinking army, the immune system is unable to carry on its routine surveillance. Frequent viral or bacterial infections may result.

Let's stop a minute and see where we are. The human in question may well present this complaint to her physician: "I feel like I'm falling apart." Over a period of time the patient has changed from a healthy, well-functioning individual to one plagued by a multitude of miseries with no obvious cause or connection. Let us examine the events and substantiate the symptoms:

Yeast overgrowth = craving sweets, starchy foods.

Yeast overgrowth = fatigue caused by undernutrition from poor absorption.

Yeast overgrowth = immune system is compromised, in disarray, ineffective.

Yeast overgrowth = constipation or diarrhea, worsening absorption, allowing yeast to proliferate.

Yeast overgrowth = the integrity of the intestinal lining is compromised, allowing abnormal-size particles of food to enter the bloodstream. Also, particles of yeast may enter the bloodstream and disseminate to other tissues.

Yeast overgrowth = disseminated yeast may compromise other organ systems, increasing demands on immune system. At some point endocrine organs may begin to malfunction, resulting in signs of autoimmune disease. The thyroid, the pancreas, adrenals, and the ovaries and gonads are affected. Weight gain reaches logarithmic growth, fueled by the sugar and starch cravings. Insulin production cannot keep up, and insulin resistance results from poor-quality insulin. Fat storage intensifies because of large amounts of sugar and insulin.

Then come the food sensitivities...

Food sensitivities = repeated exposure to food demands response of compromised immune system.

Food sensitivities = increased stress on the immune system may result in other organ malfunction due to autoimmune disease.

Food sensitivities = various symptoms develop depending on response of immune system to food. Sinus drainage, arthritis, irritable bowel, migraines, attention deficit disorder, skin rashes, eczema, depression.

Food sensitivities = intensified cravings, now for the serotonin or endorphin effect needed by the brain to tolerate the stress of total disintegration of orderly organ function. Depression may intensify from the feelings of helplessness.

At this point, assuming nothing has been done to alleviate this rapid deterioration of the immune system, other body organs begin to malfunction. These events may cause rapid aging. To justify the symptoms of food sensitivities, patients often relate that they are "just getting older." Like the proverbial toppling dominoes, the body begins to malfunction in a systematic fashion. Seemingly out of control, the reaction is actually the logical, predictable sequence of events resulting from a failure to treat the problem.

Granted, the preceding description may represent a worst-case scenario. But even if the system achieves a plateau at some point in the progression, the result is a less-than-healthy body forever destined to depend on the medical community for relief of isolated symptoms. Treating the isolated symptoms as they appear prolongs the disease. Treating the yeast and food intolerance is the answer.

Eating Has Its Limits

Many overweight patients simply love to eat. Not necessarily craving any particular food, they just don't stop eating until there is no more food. These patients assume that their digestive system simply digests everything they eat. Without regard for the fact that sensitive digestive enzymes must be made by the body ahead of time and are actually in limited supply, these people only stop eating when signaled by empty plates (theirs and those of the people sitting on either side). In these individuals food intolerance seems like a contradiction; the casual observer might think they tolerate food unusually well. In fact, these patients commonly test highly reactive to a number of foods.

These obsessive eaters enter the familiar downward spiral of health as huge excesses of food overwhelm their digestive enzymes. This results in large quantities of partially digested food entering the gut. Once in the small intestine, undigested particles of food pose a great threat if they are absorbed through the intestinal wall into the bloodstream. The immune system cells in the blood attack and destroy them but take their "fingerprint" as though they were an invading microbe. If it is an immune-mediated reaction, from that point on, the "allergic" reaction intensifies each time that food is eaten, which is frequently. The cycle is started as serotonin falls because of the allergic reaction when the reactive food is eaten. This results in further eating in an attempt to elevate the serotonin level. The process repeats itself regularly throughout the day.

Avoid overweight by eating carefully. Eat slowly. Take at least 20 minutes to finish a meal, which should consist of appropriate portions. Avoid buffets, all-you-can-eat specials, and allowing your mother to fill your plate for you. All these scenarios lend themselves to excessive portions. Chew and swallow food before taking another mouthful.

Before each bite ask yourself, "Am I still hungry?". If the answer is "No," stop eating. There is a huge caloric difference between no longer being hungry and being "full." Preserve your digestive enzymes; you only have a limited supply, and when they run out, you are done digesting and ripe for some big-time food intolerance.

Food, the Ultimate Drug

In its broadest interpretation, food must be considered a drug. Although most of us think of drugs as potent chemical formulations carefully compounded by "super smart" scientists to treat disease, this mind-set intimidates us into believing that we are not smart enough to take care of our own bodies, so we rush to seek professional help and their miracle drugs. In fact a large percentage of all drugs are derived from plants—from food, if you will (digitalis from foxglove, for example). Yes, some require extensive processing, but the fact remains that, in many cases, drugs are derived from our food. Remember that pure chocolate derived from the cocoa bean has marvelous antioxidant qualities, and sugar derived from the sugar cane, sugar beet, and corn has profound serotonin effects, as explained above. And it follows that if we can have adverse reactions to these drugs, we might also react negatively to foods. And if some drugs may have the side effects of overweight, headaches, and gastrointestinal distress, why do many of us find it unthinkable that food might do the same?

Call it unscientific, but this concept is so logical it need not wait for confirmation through medical school studies on thousands of patients; however, these studies are now being planned. Reams of existing studies, however, do allude to the influence of food on various disorders. Individually, such studies are easily ignored as isolated curiosities; but when collectively viewed as providing information about food intolerance, they take on new meaning and significance.

Food is a drug with which we dose ourselves by our eating. Foods elicit specific chemical reactions in our bodies, some to our benefit and others to our detriment. Foods by definition are foreign to the body and, like all foreign objects, have the potential to be isolated and eradicated by the immune system. To minimize this event and to allow for the orderly assimilation of nutrients, our digestive enzymes are designed to break food down into its smallest components before absorption. The immune system does not react to individual amino acids, fatty acids, or short carbon chains, which represent the smallest building blocks of proteins, fats, and carbohydrates.

To embrace the potential benefits of food and fail to recognize that food may also cause many of our ills by virtue of its chemistry is closed-minded and unscientific.

Likewise, the minerals and vitamins within our food are safely absorbed after proper digestion has freed them from the larger food macromolecule. Once past the immune system barrier, these food components may proceed through the bloodstream to be used by the body. But in the event that food is not completely digested, the immune system barrier lining in the intestine and in the bloodstream will make every effort to destroy the food as though it were a large bacterium or virus or foreign chemical. If the food macromolecule happens to pass through the intestinal lining into the bloodstream, other immune system cells continue to attack and destroy it. In the process, these immune system cells elicit the release of chemicals that have direct effects on the surrounding tissue. The resulting inflammation, swelling, and pain become the hallmark of that food in the body. Thus the healthy immune system response intended for an invading virus is mistakenly directed toward food that is eaten repeatedly and results in a series of symptoms.

Who Is That Masked Man?

The chronic nature of symptoms associated with food intolerance may be so insidious and subtle as that they are accepted as "normal." After repeatedly hearing from doctors that they will just have to live these symptoms, patients often simply accept them. However, living with chronic symptoms is unnecessary when these symptoms are related to foods that could be eliminated. The low-grade, chronic nature of a delayed food reaction is called "masking" because it conceals the food as the perpetrator. Similar to the way a hangover is "cured" by an alcoholic drink in the morning, moderate, but consistent intake of foods to which you are intolerant will temporarily alleviate "withdrawal" symptoms and thus "mask" the existence of the intolerance. Also, the chronic nature of the symptoms and the delay between eating the food and the appearance of symptoms makes it difficult to identify the specific offending food.

Unlike tedious trial elimination diets, the ALCAT test speeds the process of identifying the foods most likely at fault. In addition to identifying likely perpetrators, the ALCAT test identifies "safe" foods that elicit no reaction. These foods are useful to fall back on while you conclusively identify foods responsible for your undesirable symptoms. Examples of "mask" symptoms are fatigue, chronic sinusitis, rhinitis, arthritis, depression, colitis, and attention deficit disorder. Keep in mind that food intolerance may mimic virtually any condition or symptom.

In her 1988 book *The Food Pharmacy*, Jean Carper specifically identifies the variety of drug-like effects our foods can have on us. From apples, which lower cholesterol and blood pressure, to yogurt, which prevents ulcers and boosts the immune system, our foods are invaluable drugs to promote our health. And, like drugs, foods may elicit reactions other than those for which they are taken. The same apple that lowers your cholesterol may precipitate stomach aches and diarrhea days later. The yogurt may cause a rash on your arms. To embrace the potential benefits of food and fail to recognize that food may also cause many of our ills by virtue of its chemistry is closed-minded and unscientific.

To Be or Not to Be . . . Sick

Jean Carper and her experts predict that "eating in the future will increasingly be a therapeutic experience" and "people will come to depend more on foods and less on drugs to preserve health." This profound observation is testimony to how important it is sometimes to state the obvious. This future experience is happening now, as everyday people identify the foods that prevent them from living life to the fullest. Our future good health and happiness depends on our keen awareness of foods that keep us well and those that make us sick enough to need drugs. According to Dr. David Satcher, director of the Centers for Disease Control and Prevention, it is unacceptable that as a nation, "We only spend 1 percent of our health care budget on prevention. We tend to be crisis oriented when it comes to health." We deserve more than a food pyramid of vague suggestions to stay healthy. Our schoolchildren deserve a comprehensive curriculum so they can learn that foods can help them as well as cause their miseries. Just as they are protected from tobacco, our children should be protected from sugars and processed foods that have been stripped of nutritional value.

Because these sugars and processed grains can predispose us to food intolerance, they should be avoided. They have minimal if any nutritional value, as processing removes valuable vitamins and minerals and adds sugar in amounts toxic to the brain and immune system. Separated from their naturally valuable, healthy constituents, these simple carbohydrates now only serve to derail our efficient insulin balance, resulting in frantic storage of fat. Unfortunately, the revered food pyramid does not differentiate between whole grains and processed grains, or among fresh, frozen, and canned vegetables. And these nutritional differences can be vast. To clarify our unenviable situation, two of the largest industries in this country are the fast-food industry and the health care industry. And we pass from one to the other in assembly-line monotony.

A Drug by Any Other Name

Louise arrived at her doctor's office after local news coverage of the ALCAT test. She was 75 pounds overweight. The victim of irritable bowel syndrome for several years, she had given up taking steroid medication because it caused her to swell up so badly. She was so fatigued she often chose not to get out of bed until after noon and even then did so laboriously. Chronic sinus congestion and drainage, migraine headaches, and depression—all previously diagnosed and treated symptomatically—continually plagued her.

Despite her lack of confidence in the medical system, after she heard the newscast she felt sure that foods were her problem. Like many patients, she had already made her own diagnosis. She was food intolerant but didn't know how to go about determining which foods bothered her. After the doctor heard her story and reviewed her dietary history, she was given the ALCAT test. Before she left the office she was given instructions to avoid all "wheats and sweets" until the test results were in. Two days later she called the office to report she was feeling much better and her fatigue had disappeared. Her test results showed that she was sensitive to eggs, beef, wheat, soy, olives, and peanuts (among other foods).

Now, more convinced than ever, she began a full elimination diet in earnest. Within two weeks, every one of her symptoms had resolved with the exception of the extreme dryness of the skin on her hands. She wanted to know how long before her excess weight would come off. She was told that this would take a little longer, while she made some healthy changes in her eating habits and avoided the foods to which she was reactive.

For the first time in her adult memory, Louise was not controlled by food, bothered by a plethora of miseries leading her to overeat. She had become an exuberant schoolgirl in contrast to the defeated soul who had wandered into the office to ask about the blood test mentioned on the news. For Louise, food was a drug—a drug that precipitated bowel cramping, sinus congestion, overweight, migraine headaches, and demoralizing fatigue. Food was a drug she was willing to use with caution to avoid its devastating side effects.

Synopsis

1. Overweight is a neglected epidemic ravaging the very foundation of the American health system.

2. Government, professionals, and health care workers must rally to face the challenge posed by obesity. Health insurance must be made to cover the treatment of overweight.

3. Foods have effects on serotonin and insulin levels.

4. Intestinal overgrowth of candida yeast has a relationship to food sensitivities and cravings.

5. Food is a drug, and like drugs has side effects.

CHAPTER 6

Yo-Yo Dieting

Many misconceptions about weight loss perpetuate the very problem they purport to solve. Diet medications offer temporary appetite suppression that returns with a vengeance when the drugs are stopped. Failure to take into consideration the interrelationship of food intolerance, insulin, serotonin, and thyroid leads to many confusing and unsuccessful weight loss plans—and to what is often called "yo-yo dieting."

Yo-yo dieting has been around for a long time, but within the last 20 years it has reached national pastime proportions, probably through the popular use of appetite suppressants to speed weight loss. As their weight started going up and down faster, the descriptive term "yo-yo" captured the fancy of frustrated dieters.

"At last," they felt, "there is a name for what happens to me." True, but that is not how they seem to perceive it. Their bodies began to rapidly conserve energy when food was scarce and rapidly store energy when food was plentiful. "Yo-yoing" characterizes a predictable biologic response. In many cases, when undiscovered food sensitivities are present, the culprit food is never completely eliminated as a reactive stimulus. On discontinuing medications, dieters resume previous eating habits, often including reactive foods on a regular basis. Because the documented blood reaction to untolerated food results in a decrease in serotonin levels, dieters compensate by eating serotonin-enhancing foods. Most foods that stimulate the production of serotonin also increase insulin production, which results in several things happening in your body:

1. Blood sugar will eventually drop. When it drops below a predetermined level, you will get hungry or pass out.

2. Your fat cells will open wide and store fat voraciously, because you are obviously using blood sugar for energy and don't need the fat for energy.

3. Your fat cells will not release fat into your bloodstream to be used for energy because the glucose in your blood is a preferred energy source when it is available.

4. The production of eicosanoids (prostaglandins that are inflammatory mediators) produces allergic symptoms.

None of these events is particularly good news if you are trying to lose weight. So if we accept that the release of insulin is counterproductive to weight loss, let's identify those substances that stimulate the release of insulin into the bloodstream. Obviously, sugar in all its forms and permutations (look for items such as sucrose, fructose, dextrose, lactose, and galactose on food ingredient labels) stimulates insulin production. It's complicated to avoid just sugars!

Well, get ready for this: Refined grains may actually raise your insulin level higher and faster than sugar. If you think this includes white flour (and most anything made from it), bread, cereal, bagels, rolls, muffins, and pastries, you are right. In addition, high-sugar fruits may cause your insulin level to rise. Even the sweet taste of aspartame in your mouth causes your pancreas to start producing insulin. A large study by the American Cancer Society a few years ago yielded surprising results that received little attention. This study was to evaluate the ingestion of aspartame as a cancer risk. Although the carcinogenic effect of aspartame was inconclusive, the researchers noticed a curiosity among the participants drinking aspartame-sweetened sodas on a regular basis. These subjects gained more weight than did those who drank sugar-sweetened sodas on a regular basis.

Yo-yo dieting has been around for a long time, but within the last 20 years it has reached national pastime proportions, probably through the popular use of appetite suppressants to speed weight loss.

When the researchers studied this particular aspect in more detail, they learned that aspartame promotes a significant rise in insulin an hour or two later. Terrific, you think, now you have really faked out your body—you have all this insulin floating around with no sugar for it to work on. Remember what happens when you have low blood sugar (see item 1 in the list given earlier). That's right— you get hungry. Welcome to the merry-go-round! Now eat some sweet treat because you faithfully drank a diet drink to avoid the calories. Wait a minute—factor in the stress of juggling family, job, finances, relationships, and healthy eating. In a blink of an eye you realize that while the media had you so afraid of yo-yoing, you had actually become a one-person circus act. You are yo-yoing, juggling— and ballooning—on the merry-go-round.

It's no wonder we are confused about losing weight; even the diet food staples—bagels and diet sodas—are keeping us fat. It's as though someone gave us rules to the wrong game. Where does the madness end?

It ends with your reading books like this one and sifting through all the advertising hype. Get off the merry-go-round, put your yo-yo in your pocket, and practice juggling just two items at a time before throwing everything into the air at once. Go back to basics: Drink filtered water and eat basic foods—vegetables, fruits, and meats. Shun the fancy gourmet knock-off that slathers the food with sugar and fat, freezes it, then boasts that it tastes good and is good for you. Get smart, buy a steamer, and cook up a batch of fresh veggies. To control your weight, relinquish sugars and refined grains. Learn to identify and avoid foods that cause a rapid rise in insulin. These are typically foods that you will crave as a result of eating your allergic foods. A fairly complete list of these foods can be found in *The G-Index Diet* (1993) by Richard Podell, M.D. If you think you may suffer from food sensitivities, intestinal candidiasis, or subclinical hypothyroidism, see a physician who will help you decide the best way to diagnose and treat these problems.

If the stress of everyday life is contributing to your weight gain, see a physician who recognizes and promotes stress management and lifestyle adjustment programs as a valuable part of weight control. The point is, don't rush out and take appetite suppressants, herbs, or 90-day wonder cures for weight loss. Understand that something is wrong and it can be treated rather then covered up.

If Yo-Yoing Is Bad, Why Not Stay Fat?

Overweight and obesity dramatically increase the risk of the serious diseases of diabetes, hypertension, stroke, gall bladder disease, arthritis, breast, prostate, and colon cancer, and cardiovascular disease. Of these the most devastating is Type 2 diabetes. This is because Type 2 or so-called adult onset diabetes is directly related to overweight and as such is almost entirely preventable. There are about 15 million diabetics in the United States and about 90 percent of these are Type 2 diabetics. Diabetes has been shown to be directly related to BMI (body mass index). That is, the heavier one gets the more likely he or she is to eventually become diabetic. A study by Mokdad and colleagues and associates, examining the trends in diabetes prevalence in the United States between 1990 and 2000, revealed a parallel increase in the incidence of obesity. From 1999 to 2000 the average American adult weight increased by 0.5 kilograms and the risk of diabetes increased by about 6 percent. Previous data revealed that for every 2.2 pounds of weight increase, the risk of diabetes increases by 9 percent. Stop here a moment and think about a friend or family member with diabetes and the heartbreak associated with this disease, not to mention the significantly shortened life span. And for the most part it is entirely preventable by losing weight and keeping it off.

It is very important to understand that one need not lose down to one's ideal weight to benefit. In "The Role of Weight Loss in Improving Metabolic Outcomes," F. Xavier Pi-Sunyer, M.D., on Medscape's Web site reported that a modest weight loss of 5 to 10 percent of body weight is associated with a 58 percent decrease in incidence of diabetes, and significant improvements in blood pressure, lipid levels and mortality. Weight loss results in improved glycemic control and insulin sensitivity. Overall, it is a no-brainer. The bad news is that overweight and obesity cause diabetes, the good news is that by losing weight you can stop this from happening. Forget that the IRS may let you deduct the cost of weight loss. Do it because you want to live a long and disease-free life. I believe pretty much all of you have figured out that you don't want to spend much time in doctor's offices or hospitals—so lose the weight, stop yo-yoing around.

Who Came Up with This Food Pyramid, Anyhow?

It is interesting that the official USDA food pyramid recommends a large sampling of grains and fruit each day. This pyramid may represent a way to assure adequate nutrient intake in the form of vitamins and minerals, but it certainly is no way to lose weight. Whereas the USDA food pyramid was not intended as a with loss plan a normal healthy eating should promote normal weight. As noted by Dr. Barry Sears in his book *The Zone,* the food pyramid closely resembles the proportions of fat, protein, and carbohydrates fed to cattle in feedlots to fatten them for slaughter. I suggest you rethink the food pyramid. If it fattens cattle so well, why would it make us thinner? Observe that "food pyramid" Americans aren't getting thinner; they are getting fatter. And that's not just a coincidence.

The 2001 Annual Meeting of the North American Association for the Study of Obesity revealed preliminary results from a three-center study comparing the Adkins high-protein diet to a conventional low-fat, high-carbohydrate plan. The researchers concluded that the Adkins diet produced favorable results on weight, HDL (High Density Lipoproteins, a combination of fat and proteins which carry cholesterol from the cells to the liver for breakdown and elimination from the body), triglycerides (the main type of stored fats in animals), and retention of study subjects. The low-fat plan showed favorable effects on total cholesterol and LDL (Low Density Lipoprotein cholesterol is commonly referred to as "bad cholesterol") and is thought to be a major risk factor for heart disease cholesterol. Lose the pyramid, folks, it's a bust. And to make your diet work even better, determine your food sensitivities and lock out the processed grains and sweets.

Processed Foods:
Are All Carbohydrates Created Equal?

Grains are nutritionally great for you—when they are whole-grain products and only when you are not sensitive to them. Whole-grain foods are not rare; they are just rarely eaten. Most grains we eat in this country have been so highly processed and adulterated that one might safely conclude their only value lies in name recognition for advertising. Overusing and overeating processed foods such as highly refined grains predisposes us to developing food sensitivities. Much is missing from this nutritionally dead food. Regardless of how much synthetic nutrient is put back in after processing, the food has changed form and cannot substitute for the natural form.

But no matter how nutritionally worthless the processed food may be to the body, it can still stimulate the digestive system. Your digestive system doesn't realize you haven't the sense to avoid worthless food; it trusts that you intentionally ate this high-starch, high-sugar, and high-fat meal for a good reason. After all, you are the one with the brain.

At the expense of untold quantities of digestive enzymes, your digestive system scrounges every available nutrient from this barren wasteland, void of vitamins and minerals, called processed food. Foraging, as it will, the body is able to glean carbohydrates, fats, and a few proteins from this synthetic food. Even the synthetic vitamins that "fortify" it may defy identification and use by the body. Because all the useful enzymes were removed during processing, your body must enzymatically finance this digestive venture. But to avoid being entirely pessimistic, your pancreas responds admirably to the rise in blood sugar brought on by the processed carbohydrate that has no other nutritional value. As a result, all that nutritionally worthless fat that had been added to the processed grain to make it palatable now has set up permanent residence on your hips, thighs, and buttocks. (Maybe that's why they call it a food pyramid! If we eat what they tell us to, we will resemble a pyramid!)

So despite all the hope your digestive system puts into processing each meal, many meals are simply bad investments. All in all, the body must use up enzymes and hormones that are more valuable than the little nutrient available in the food.

Medications and Weight Loss: How Long Can This Go On?

Prescription medications for weight loss have become a lucrative profit center for large pharmaceutical companies. The basic deficiency of current weight loss medications lies in the fact that they are explicitly intended for the relief of symptoms (hunger). The treatment of overweight should not be confused with the treatment of hunger, which is what prescribing medicine is about. Although a common symptom of overweight patients, hunger is by no means the underlying cause of their overweight. Inappropriate hunger doesn't just happen; chemical changes in the body result in hunger. Resolving the symptom without diligent investigation as to the underlying cause is tantamount to teasing the patient into thinking the disease is cured. Once the medications are no longer prescribed, the unresolved or unidentified etiology of the overweight re-emerges, resulting in weight regain.

The good news is that when your reactive foods are eliminated, your problem with overweight slowly disappears and remains gone.

The main point to establish here is that the medications whether they be appetite suppressants, fat blockers, or antidepressants only work as long as you take them. If you are overweight, it happened because of an aberration in your biochemistry, not because you had low blood levels of these drugs. So if you aren't finding and fixing the problem while you are taking medication, you are doomed to yo-yo back up in weight when you stop the drugs. Unlike drug therapy, avoidance of incompatible foods normalizes your metabolism, which should remain so, provided there is no other endocrine disease. Therefore, when your reactive foods are eliminated, your problem with overweight slowly disappears, and remains gone.

Further, all current medications are indicated only for relatively short periods of time. Because most studies are only done for limited periods, the medication is approved for only that time frame. If in that period of time a reasonable cause and treatment has not been established for the overweight problem, the patient would seem to be out of luck. It would be up to the discretion of the physician to extend treatment past the time approved.

Thus, short-term treatment of weight problems with drug therapy is similar to treating the diabetic patient with insulin for the symptom of high blood sugar. They are both long-term problems, unless the underlying cause is addressed. If we removed the insulin, the blood sugar values would surely begin showing symptoms of high blood sugar. Unless a specific remedy to renew the pancreas's ability to produce insulin is instituted and the cells regain sensitivity to the insulin that is produced, the underlying disease is not cured and treatment must continue. Because no one has become overweight from a deficiency of appetite suppressant in the blood, it stands to reason that appetite suppressant should only be used with the intention of giving symptomatic relief while the true disease is investigated and treated. So, unless the underlying cause of metabolic imbalance is addressed by implementing appropriate dietary change, short term drug interventions only worsen matters.

Am I Really Hungry?

Granted, hunger is a contributing factor to the development of overweight. More important to the cure of overweight is the underlying drive to eat, which the patient interprets as hunger. Why do some people feel "hungry" at inappropriate times? First, I believe our discussion will benefit from a technically correct definition. "Hunger" as defined by Webster's dictionary is "a strong desire or need for food." In the overweight patient, "need" and "desire" for food are two very different feelings. Need implies supplying nutrient required to sustain life. Desire for food, in contrast, implies satisfaction of a wish, a dream, a pleasure if you will. Satisfying the *need* for food would seem to carry little risk of incidental excess calories as nutritional deficiencies of the body are satisfied, but satisfying the *desire* for food carries the risks of reckless abandon as one eats to satisfy a much more ephemeral calling. Without regard for nutrients, one may consume food to ease the pain of chemical imbalances created by mental, psychological, or physiological stress. Incredible sums of unneeded calories may be consumed to alleviate stress-lowered serotonin levels, or to satiate proliferating yeast.

Nonetheless, appetite suppressants relieve hunger defined as the desire or need for food. Now if you take appetite suppressants to let you evaluate and select wise food choices that minimize unnecessary caloric intake and maximize nutrient intake, you eliminate the incidental calories by eating needed food. If you take appetite suppressants to indiscriminately reduce the amount of food you eat, you may well precipitate nutrient deficiencies in your body. These in turn will result in hunger defined as the need for nutrient. A vicious cycle of gross proportions ensues.

How Should I Eat?

Appetite suppressants should be used only to allow individuals to make wise food choices, never to simply eat less food. Anyone taking appetite suppressants should seek professional guidance for proper nutrition. To assume that the overweight patient will make wise food choices because he isn't hungry is like assuming that an addict will write a master's thesis because he's gotten his drug fix. In both cases, the relief of physiologic symptoms does not make up for lack of education.

The overweight person must be taught how to properly nourish his or her body. To simply praise and rave over the consumption of fewer calories with no attention to life-giving nutrients is naive. A general understanding of the nutritional needs of your own body, including its food sensitivities, is imperative. You should also have a general understanding of various foods and their benefits and potential risks. You must then learn how to deal appropriately with the emotional stresses that result in your inappropriate eating.

Without intense remedial education in these areas, dieters are likely to eat less food only for a period, to satisfy a short-term goal. Weight regain is expected and predictable in those who don't know how not to regain weight. Using appetite suppressants without making a diligent effort to determine the underlying cause of your overweight and without seeking the knowledge you need to correct your deficiencies is an injustice. Having said that, let me also say that any medically supervised weight control program is a partnership. It is incumbent on both partners to do their fair share. Even the best intentions of the medical professional cannot impose weight loss on an individual unwilling to make changes in eating behavior or lifestyle.

FDA approval of appetite suppressants or drugs for weight management becomes almost a moot point when one realizes the inherent risks of any medication. In the summer 1995 edition of *Health & Wellness Today,* Dr. Julian Whitaker states, "FDA approved drugs kill 140,000 people per year! That's seven times more than die from heroin, crack, and all other illegal drugs put together!"

Taking appetite suppressants, fat binders, or metabolism enhancers without an overall program of food sensitivity testing, lifestyle modification, education, stress therapy, or diagnosis of the underlying cause of the overweight is like getting in a taxi, starting the meter, and going nowhere. You will pay a lot of money to end up exactly where you started. There are no shortcuts in the treatment of overweight, just as there are none in the treatment of diabetes, cancer, or congestive heart failure.

Fingerprinting Your Foods

As you repeatedly eat and overeat processed food, you may eventually exceed the capabilities of your digestive enzymes. This results in undigested or partially digested food in the intestine. The area of the intestine where absorption takes place is beyond the point at which digestion takes place. If undigested or partially digested food continues through the intestine, it is more likely to be absorbed as large food particles rather than the beneficial amino acids, fatty acids, and short carbon chains that can be used from the bloodstream with little modification.

Normally the wall of the intestine is highly selective about the size of particles it will absorb. However, if the wall of the gut is inflamed by viral infection, allergic response to food, candida yeast infestation, pregnancy, alcohol consumption, or any of a multitude of causes, it may absorb larger-than-normal-size food particles.

Once this larger particle of food has made it through the intestinal lining, it is for all practical purposes in the blood vessel. Here it comes under the close scrutiny of specialized immune system cells, whose job is to patrol the bloodstream watching for potential troublemakers. As these cells chemically identify the food particle, they also send off chemical signals that attract more immune system cells to the area. Eventually the food particle is neutralized and disassembled into its smallest chemical units—which, interestingly, is the exact process that the digestive enzymes should have performed in the stomach and intestine.

Just as many car accidents could be avoided by people driving slower and paying more attention, so could people avoid many food sensitivities by eating slower and paying more attention to food choices. As you see, the body has set up an excellent backup system to prevent large unidentified particles from roaming around the bloodstream, whether they are viruses, bacteria, or food. And as it does with viruses and bacteria, the immune system memorizes the chemical fingerprint of the food. In the future, anytime it sees that "fingerprint" again, it will attack the substance with even greater vigor as a repeated "threat" to the body.

Familiarity Leads to Contempt

Let's just say that the food to which you have now become sensitive (when you eat it, your immune system reacts to it in an ever-increasing intensity) happens to be one you eat every day. Perhaps it's milk, or wheat, or corn. Over a period of time the violent immune reaction to the food will result in more and more local tissue response in an attempt to isolate this invader from the rest of the body. As this "allergic reaction" spreads to surrounding tissues, the symptoms you have will represent the swelling and diminished function of body organ systems. When the lining of your colon swells up because of a food you ate, abdominal cramps and diarrhea may fill your day. If the food stimulates a response in the stomach, expect the fires of "acid reflux" to flare. If the allergic food makes it into your bloodstream, you may experience the misery of anything from "sinus congestion" to migraine headaches to skin rashes and "arthritis." This great "mockingbird of disease" may have you taking a fistful of different medications and thinking that you "are falling apart." Until you consider food as a cause of your misery, you may finance many cars and swimming pools for conventional medical practitioners.

So now you have a clearer picture of the mechanism by which indigestion, irritable bowel, colitis, and malabsorption are related to food sensitivities. Over a period of time, the immune response may signal a perpetual state of high alert as you continue to eat the same foods. Soon enough the immune system's demands for nutrients will exceed your digestive system's now-compromised ability to process and absorb nutrients.

Food Sensitivities, the Immune System, and the Thyroid

Once you have a food sensitivity, your immune system goes into hyperdrive to protect you from this persistent "invader." Over time, whether from malnutrition or just plain overactivity, your immune system goes a little haywire. It gets confused and misfires, and may even attack body parts because it can no longer distinguish between good and bad cells. This is bad enough when it results in arthritis (a common symptom associated with food sensitivities), but gets serious when it involves the thyroid.

Autoimmune destruction of the thyroid leads to decreased production of thyroid hormone. Autoimmune disease and subsequent hypothyroidism are sometimes discovered following a pregnancy. Curiously, food intolerance commonly develops during pregnancy as well. Researchers are investigating the effect of subclinical hypothyroidism on the other endocrine organs. This hypothyroidism may be the result of autoimmune destruction of part of the thyroid gland and may result in elevated insulin levels, elevated cholesterol, ovarian hormone dysfunction, depression, and weight gain due to lowered basal metabolic rate (the thyroid determines metabolic rate).

A prominent researcher in this field, Dr. Broda O. Barnes, gives an excellent review in his book *Hypothyroidism: The Unsuspected Illness* (1976). To condense the excellent treatment he gives this disease process in his book would be presumptuous. Suffice it to say that the thyroid blood tests commonly used today may not give a true picture of your thyroid function. If you are cold all the time; have a high cholesterol level; or suffer from menstrual irregularities, depression, hypertension, fatigue, and unexplained overweight, you would be well served by reading the book. Take it along as you seek a doctor who will treat you as a person rather than a blood test. There is no greater insult than to hear that because the blood test is normal, nothing is wrong; it's all in your mind. It makes one want to ask, "Well, doctor, if nothing is wrong, will you ask the blood test why I keep getting fatter, more tired, and colder?"

There are distinct relationships among food sensitivities, intestinal candidiasis, and hypothyroidism. The symptoms of each are similar and overlapping. The conditions can and should be treated separately, but until the food sensitivities are treated, nagging symptoms will persist.

How do food sensitivities keep you fat? The exact mechanism may never be known, but whether the allergic reaction makes fat inaccessible or whether it slows the thyroid is immaterial. The fact is that you have at your disposal the solution: Stop eating your allergic foods. The good news is that when your reactive foods are eliminated, your problem with overweight slowly disappears. Side effects of general well-being, clearing of the mind, and more energy lead to the opportunity to exercise and ultimately there is no better way to assure weight loss than to exercise while avoiding your reactive foods. Feel good, look good, life is good.

An inflammatory response occurs in the bloodstream following the absorption of a reactive food. Presumably this inflammatory or "allergic reaction" has the potential to damage local organs and tissues if the reaction is prolonged or intense enough. Certainly this reaction consumes large amounts of nutrients and energy as the immune network of the body struggles to protect us from our food.

With time the immune system becomes more frantic as it senses it cannot control the invading organism (food). Decreasing nutritional absorption, increasing demands on immune cells, and limitations imposed on the immune system by stress hormones result in anarchy in the immune network. Much like soldiers revolting against tyranny, the immune system begins to attack the endocrine organs, as well as other body tissues. Of the organs most susceptible and sensitive to autoimmune disease, the thyroid, the pancreas, and the ovaries appear to have a major influence on our weight. Many women experience thyroiditis (thyroid inflammation) following pregnancy, which may later result in a lowering of thyroid function. We also know that food sensitivities can result in autoimmune damage to organs and that pregnancy is a common time to develop food sensitivities.

This development probably results from disturbances of gastrointestinal function and absorption related to hormonal changes associated with pregnancy. Not only does the thyroid control the body's metabolic rate through the hormones it secretes, but it also affects the other endocrine organs and the hormones they secrete as well. For example, as thyroid hormone levels drop, the effect on the pancreas is to increase insulin secretion and the effect on the liver is to increase cholesterol levels and stimulate the conversion of carbohydrates to fat for storage.

Changes in thyroid hormone levels may have seemingly irrational effects on ovarian hormone production. These fluctuating hormone levels result in menstrual irregularities and premenopausal symptoms that often defy treatment. Treating these symptoms is difficult, because it is like trying to hit a moving target as the hormone levels fluctuate wildly in response to erratic thyroid hormone levels from the sick or failing thyroid. Some degree of control is possible if one does not depend on the usual thyroid blood tests as the unequivocal measure of thyroid hormone activity at the cellular level. This brings to mind the book *Living Well with Hypothyroidism* by Mary Shomon. She also has a very informative Web site at www.thyroid.about.com. Mary was one of thousands of women who suffer from untreated hypothyroidism. Her doctors would not treat her because her blood tests showed no abnormality. Her story, in-depth discussion, and useful instructions of how to help your doctor to make the diagnosis is a testimony to my belief that you don't have to be a member of the exclusive Doctors' Club to understand your body and to do something about it.

Body Temperature
Tells the Thyroid Story

The current blood tests we have for evaluating thyroid function are much better screening tests than those available in the past. But using a screening test to evaluate the true effect of thyroid hormone on its end organ cells does not make good sense. As we all know, quality and quantity are very different measurements and must not be confused. At this point one is not questioning whether a certain level of hormone is available in the blood or not. We need to know whether the level of thyroid hormone in the blood is adequately stimulating the appropriate cells and adequately maintaining an appropriate metabolic rate.

One simple way to evaluate clinically the effect of thyroid hormone is to monitor your basal body temperature. For all practical purposes (barring fever, illness, or effects of drugs), the basal body temperature reflects the metabolic activity and clinically correlates closely with thyroid hormone function.

The first mistake is trying to treat symptoms to affect a cure. Symptoms should be used to help identify the problem; treatment should be directed at solving the problem. Symptoms are alleviated at the discretion of a compassionate physician. Treatment, in contrast, is a commitment, a partnership, a goal-oriented effort to improve quality of life through the correction of inborn or self-induced deficiencies in body functions. The point is that the job is simply not done until the cause of the symptoms is corrected.

If you took your car to a mechanic because it was making a noise and he told you to turn the radio up and the noise would go away, I doubt you would feel confident that your problem had been solved. But how many of us leave our doctor's office with medicine to cover up the signs of our diseases of overweight, hypertension, diabetes, and menstrual irregularities? Like the figurative ostrich sticking its head in the sand, we may believe that if we don't see a problem, it doesn't exist. Well, if you don't look for a problem, you will never see it. The "body mechanics" who identify and eliminate food sensitivity offer the limitless rewards of a fully functional reconditioned body with a renewed factory-serviced warranty.

Most importantly, keep in mind that even after you have your computer serviced, you still must decide which programs to load to serve your needs best. You may still have work to do regarding the various chronic conditions influenced by food sensitivities. At least you have "fixed the computer" by eliminating your reactive foods. Thyroid, insulin, and serotonin will be freed from the influence of food intolerance, and eating and exercising right will show further results in weight loss.

Synopsis

1. Weight regain or yo-yoing after weight loss is a predictable event based on food sensitivities, hormones, and survival genes.

2. Close review of the "food pyramid" raises questions.

3. Prescription medications to aid in weight loss have a limited and well-defined value, allowing temporary support while the underlying cause of overweight is dealt with.

4. Food sensitivities, thyroid malfunction, candida yeast, and immune system disease may all play a role in weight gain and other mysterious symptoms. They all defy identification and are often overlooked by conventional medicine.

5. Food sensitivities can be accurately determined with the ALCAT test; thyroid and candida issues are treatable with the assistance of a knowledgable health practitioner.

CHAPTER 7

Food Intolerance: The Missed Diagnosis

Virtually every human who comes to recognize food sensitivities as the source of their physical ailments feels as though their story is unique and incredible. We are so indoctrinated that foods cannot be the cause of our misery that we feel as though we are a medical wonder. In fact, we may be nothing more than the misinformed majority.

My Story

I can't say the exact day it happened, but I can tell you it felt like the floor disappeared from under me. The day I realized that food intolerance was responsible for my obesity, my attitude toward medicine changed. For almost 20 years as a physician, I had pretty much accepted the conventional mind-set. I treated symptoms and treated them well, sometimes over and over again in the same patient. Nonetheless my patients' gratitude satisfied my ego as they acknowledged me as a good and caring physician. Despite my caring demeanor, I had an intense dread of treating overweight patients. I was frustrated that these patients could not understand—their overweight interfered with my treatment.

Actually I was frustrated by my inability to treat their overweight successfully, because what I knew about treating obesity was woefully inadequate. Because it seemed only a matter of willpower to push away from the table, I chastised them for not simply eating less. I now apologize to all these patients. You were ill and, because I didn't know how to help you, I passed the blame. I know now that you had no more control over your eating than the diabetic has over his pancreas.

My professional existence at the time was based on my extensive knowledge (memorizing) of chemical concoctions. These relieved symptoms until the body could cure itself. In my later practice years I depended entirely on the use of chemicals as an anesthesiologist. Even in this profession I dreaded the overweight patient for the increased risks imposed. Obesity, an illness for which I had not learned a treatment, was an affront to my skill as a doctor.

Not until I caught the disease and faced the monster myself did I appreciate the devastating effect obesity has on the quality of life.

My own health began to deteriorate the year my daughter was born and my wife was diagnosed with breast cancer. My wife died a year and a half after our daughter's birth. Then circumstances beyond my control forced me to seek other job opportunities. Meanwhile, my health continued to deteriorate over the years as my weight increased steadily through another marriage and a divorce. I was disgusted by my weight—245 pounds on a 5'9" frame. Job stress increased, and I became unable to adequately care for my eight-year-old daughter and fulfill my responsibilities as a medical school anesthesiology instructor. I was a mess.

It is not uncommon to crave the very food to which you are sensitive.

At the time of my divorce I decided to change my life. I lost 45 pounds in a physician-supervised weight-loss program using medication. Feeling redeemed and enlightened by having trimmed down, I resigned my medical school instructor position and began the necessary studies to become board-certified in bariatric medicine the following year. I opened my own medical weight management office. My health was recovering and job stress was much reduced. Nutritional supplements and healthy eating habits were making all the difference. When I opened my own office, I had maintained my 200-pound weight for about six months. Not thin, but stabilized at a weight I found acceptable.

I first learned about food intolerance at a medical conference. Curious about the relationship of food intolerance to overweight, I had the ALCAT Test run on myself. I was about to go through the most rapid growth spurt of my professional life. I can remember shaking my head when I looked at my test results—positive to corn, wheat, tomatoes, beans, peppers, and turkey among other things. It baffled me to think that these "healthy" foods could contribute to my overweight problem. Most of them had, in fact, been staples of my recent successful weight loss. Nonetheless, I made the commitment and was determined to see it through.

I attacked the elimination of corn and wheat at the same time, and soon learned that 75 percent of the packaged goods at the grocery store contain corn or corn products. Wheat, on the other hand, turned up in the ingredients of all sorts of cereals, snacks, frozen entrees, and breads. Regular trips to a local health-food store became routine. Things started to fall into place once I became a dedicated label reader. Without realizing it, I had become addicted to corn and wheat. Fortunately, there are many acceptable substitutes for wheat and corn. In fact, a whole subculture of enlightened individuals who scorn traditional grocery stores are turning instead to merchants who offer wide varieties of organic produce and alternatives to common grains.

The other vegetables and the meat to which I was sensitive were easier to avoid. I distributed the peppers, tomatoes, and beans in my robust garden that year to family and friends, and changed my eating habits. After a couple months I became pleasantly aware that my craving for sweets had disappeared. My daughter could actually make her chocolate chip cookies and not worry that they would disappear while she was at school. Most remarkably, my weight resumed its downward spiral. I became more alert and had more energy than I'd had since college. I felt alive now that fatigue was no longer part of my daily existence. It was as though the accumulation of years of digestive sediment and barnacles of malnutrition had been scraped away.

Surprisingly, after the first difficult two weeks, I don't remember any discomfort from cravings or hunger. As long as I only ate when I was hungry and avoided my reactive foods, I ate whatever I wanted and lost weight each week. That's not to say that I ate what others may have wanted me to eat, but using basic common sense in avoiding fats and sugars, I lost weight effortlessly to the 175-pound range I have maintained for over a year now. I didn't have a nutrition degree, food scale, stair stepper, Richard Simmons tape, or nasty-tasting diet-in-a-can. I really did eat what I wanted; I just didn't want a lot of the unhealthy foods as long as I avoided my reactive foods.

How Do You Know When You React to a Food?

One particular episode comes to mind. My daughter and I, late for a school function, decided to grab something fast to eat on the way. Because of my food sensitivities I was preparing most of our meals because restaurants tend to mix foods for flavor, making it unrealistic for me to eat out and stay on my elimination diet. Nevertheless, we stopped at a fast-food restaurant and, for some reason, the picture of a hot bowl of chili called to me. I'm not particularly fond of chili, but food sensitivities do funny things to your mind. It is not uncommon to crave the very food to which you are sensitive.

At any rate, halfway through the bowl of chili I thought, "This has to have tomatoes in it." In a minor panic I stopped eating. It had been two full weeks since I had eaten tomatoes. About an hour later, a half-hour into the school program, I was overwhelmed with an intense headache and fatigue. I could not force my eyes to stay open to watch the program. Thankfully we made it through the program and got home safely. (Because driver fatigue is a cause of numerous accidents, I wonder how many food-sensitivity victims fall asleep at the wheel.)

I had learned a valuable lesson to pass on to my patients. Make the commitment to eliminate the food that causes you unpleasant symptoms and you will be held to that commitment. I had reneged on my commitment by unintentionally eating tomatoes in the chili. My immune system soon recognized this almost-forgotten "invader" and attacked it in a hyper-acute response. This premature reintroduction of a reactive food after a period of elimination resulted in a rapid deployment of immune system soldier cells. These cells along with the chemical reactions they elicited in the surrounding cells brought about headache, fuzzy thinking, fatigue, and runny nose. This personal experience brought to my reality a dramatic event I had only read about.

Must I Forever Forsake My Favorite Foods?

I have since reintroduced all my reactive foods into my diet. I know I cannot eat turkey without developing fatigue, and that cooked tomatoes will give me a headache. I realize my limits, and life is good when I respect these limitations.

Although classical allergy reactions are pretty much permanent, in the case of food sensitivities, remove the food for a period of time and the body often forgives and forgets. Commonly after a period of three months, reintroducing the food is worthwhile. If it elicits no immediate reaction, the food can be rotated through your diet about every four days with little likelihood that you'll become sensitive to it again.

Some foods simply aren't worth the trouble. One patient expressed this opinion when reminded that she could reintroduce corn to her diet. In encouraging her to overcome the difficulties in eliminating corn from her diet, I had vividly educated her in all the digestive vagaries and ill-effects associated with corn and corn products. Apparently I had been quite convincing. When I suggested she try corn again, she responded as though I had offered her poison, politely saying: "I don't think so."

Case Studies

The following histories of patients suffering from food intolerance gives some insight into the wide variety of chronic conditions amenable to cure by eliminating reactive foods. In the following case presentations, certain identifying characteristics have been changed to protect patient privacy. The stories, however, are true.

Chronic and Neglected

One cannot experience a more empathetic moment than while performing a physical examination on an overweight female patient with chronic sinus drainage, a diagnosis of irritable bowel syndrome, hypothyroidism, and depression. She evokes compassion not so much because of her individual diseases, but because she represents a neglected human contingent. This group of people has been over-treated and under-cured by conventional medicine. Instructed that they will have to live with the limitations of their "chronic disease," these patients withdraw from the spotlight of society. They survive in solitude in the shadow of their former lives.

This poor woman had been shuttled between medical specialists like a hockey puck. After each extensive exam, she was told confidently that everything checked out okay and they could find nothing wrong. Each specialist—ENT (ear, nose, and throat), endocrinologist, gastroenterologist, and psychiatrist—succeeded only in proving he or she didn't know why the woman had her symptoms. But appropriate prescription medication would take care of her discomfort. Frustrated, she turned even more frequently to her one solace—her favorite foods. Not surprisingly, her symptoms persisted, and she was led to believe she would need medication the rest of her life.

Gladys, at the age of 56, had conceded she would never lead a normal life. She was seeking help for overweight—which was ruining her life—out of desperation. Her sinus and bowel problems and depression could be covered up with medication, but her weight blatantly called attention to her despair and humiliation. She desperately wanted someone who would treat her obesity with dignity.

When asked about her weight, her desperation poured out. To the point of tears, she shook her head violently and blurted out, "I just don't know what else to do! I watch what I eat, but I just keep getting bigger." Although she was calorie-conscious and carefully avoided sugars and fats, she ate an abundance of processed carbohydrates. She had noticed that milk caused stomach pains and fatigue, so she avoided it. All Gladys's symptoms showed up on the list of common symptoms associated with food intolerance. Because of her history, we decided to perform the ALCAT Test to see whether she had other food intolerances of which she was unaware.

Years of endless defeat had led her to make her own diagnosis, one that had eluded all the specialists she had consulted. She instantly knew that her body was reacting to a food or foods. That was why no one could find anything wrong; nothing *was* wrong where they were looking. Her entire problem was hidden in her own blood vessels and in the lining of her intestine, where her cells were violently attacking food particles as though they were foreign viruses or bacteria. She could not access her fat stores for energy because of the perpetual chemical reaction that paralyzed the breakdown of her fat for energy.

To have any energy at all, she had to eat more food because her vast warehouse of energy was locked. Her immune system was frazzled by poor nutrient absorption through a gut wall swollen from reaction to her food. This crippled immune system was misfiring and the auto-immune diseases of hypothyroidism and arthritis probably represented its attacking the body itself. This avalanche of disease probably began with the absorption of poorly digested food into the bloodstream from the intestine.

Just because fitness gurus proclaim a low-calorie food "healthy" doesn't make it so.

Just because fitness gurus proclaim a low-calorie food "healthy" doesn't make it so. Each food can have a totally individual and different relationship with each person. To cure many chronic illnesses, the doctor must consider food and its potential for disease in each patient. This time-consuming and dedicated approach is beyond the scope of our current "ten-minute visit" medical system. Long forgotten are the words of Hippocrates, the father of medicine: "Let thy food be thy medicine."

Happily, Gladys underwent the ALCAT food sensitivity test, and her symptoms began to resolve quickly after her elimination diet and vitamin and mineral supplements began. Her depression lifted, her irritable bowel calmed, and her sinuses cleared quickly; she now only suffers from an occasional seasonal sinus congestion. We postponed the prescription of appetite suppressants until we saw the results of the food-elimination program: four pounds lost during the first week. She now knew which foods she could not eat.

While she remained on the food-elimination diet, she continued to lose an average of two pounds per week. After losing 21 pounds, her weight had stabilized. She now felt in control of her destiny. Although she may still make an occasional poor food selection, she makes informed choices and knows the consequences; she is finally beginning to understand and make peace with her body.

We also decided to monitor her basal body temperature to evaluate thyroid function. Over a ten-day period her basal temperature averaged 3 degrees below normal. This, along with her continuing morning fatigue, dry skin and hair, and cold intolerance suggested subclinical hypothyroidism. We reviewed the options with her and she elected to try low-dose thyroid supplementation. After two months it was hard to recognize her as the same woman who had come looking for help with her weight. She was now an alert, involved member of the human race. Her basal body temperatures were rising toward normal and her clinical thyroid blood tests remained in the normal range. With time and continued attention to avoiding her reactive foods, she may be able to decrease her thyroid medication in the future—a successful outcome considering that all she wanted in the first place was diet pills.

Fibromyalgia in a Medical Professional

A 45-year-old medical professional came to me for treatment of overweight. Very dedicated, she had successfully lost weight using medication. On her initial visit she had mentioned other physical problems, including fibromyalgia that at times was debilitating. Studies into food allergies and intolerances had revealed a possible food connection to fibromyalgia. This patient was informed about this possibility and was willing to give it a try.

She had the ALCAT Test performed. She found the results very interesting and dedicated herself to quickly eliminating her reactive foods from her diet. In short order (about two weeks), she experienced significant improvement in her condition. After a few more weeks her fibromyalgia, from which she had suffered for years, was completely resolved.

After a few months she experienced a relapse. Careful questioning revealed that she had unintentionally reintroduced some of her reactive foods. With stringent elimination of those foods, she again experienced relief of her symptoms. Through her own trial and error, she was soon able to confirm that if she ate corn in any form, her fibromyalgia returned; she also discovered that tomatoes caused her gastrointestinal discomfort. She was now in control. Even though at times she chose to eat these foods, she knew the resulting symptoms were no mystery. Knowing their cause made her symptoms less intimidating, and her ability to control their occurrence allowed her a freedom she had not known for years.

ALCAT Test Confirms Food Sensitivities

One 42-year-old male patient had been under the care of his physician for several years for overweight. He had been successful at losing 20 pounds and keeping it off. He simply went once a month to see his doctor, who gave him a prescription for Fen-Phen. Following the removal of Fenfluramine from the market, his doctor would no longer treat him for overweight.

On his first visit to a new doctor, after reviewing his history, the doctor asked if he might be interested in trying a different approach to maintaining his weight. He was open to the idea of not taking medication if he could keep his weight off without it. He had the ALCAT Test done, and the results were impressive to him. He was reactive to milk, corn, and wheat among other foods.

After discovering his reactive foods, he related that he had once passed out after eating two mouthfuls of ice cream, which contains both milk and corn. He had apparently had a pretty intense reaction to both and should eliminate them. Going down the list of his reactive foods, he confirmed that most were foods that he enjoyed daily while successfully losing his excess weight taking medication. These foods were a time bomb waiting to explode as soon as he stopped taking medication. By eliminating these foods he would be able to avoid his historic rapid weight regain.

He was also introduced to the concept of food rotation so he would not eat the same foods more than once every four days. This would allow his body to process and clear the innocent mistakes made by his immune system as it continued trying to protect his body from perceived invaders. He welcomed the opportunity to stop taking medication and still keep his weight off.

Attention-Deficit Disorder and Sugar Intolerance

A 13-year-old girl was brought to the office following a news broadcast of the potential benefits of eliminating reactive foods in the treatment of ADD. At an early age she had been put on Ritalin and other medication for ADD at the recommendation of teachers and doctors. After giving her medication for a couple of years, her parents decided to stop. The little girl confirmed that the medicine made her feel "funny" and she didn't like it. She also admitted that she didn't like it when her mind wandered and she forgot to do things she was supposed to do. She said she could not help it and found it embarrassing.

She related that school was becoming more and more difficult and she had received her first "F." In addition to her ADD, she had suffered from recurrent ear infections when she was younger and had strange itchy skin rashes that would come and go. One on her right leg remained itchy and scaly. Her sinus drainage problems were a constant sniffing, coughing presence. Her eating history was loaded with sugar. Interestingly, a good bit of the sugar in her diet came with the blessing of the school that diagnosed her with ADD, resulting in years of medication. After a heart-to-heart talk with mother and daughter regarding the immediate elimination of all sugars and corn products from the girl's diet, she had the ALCAT Test done, which confirmed her intolerance to sugar and corn.

In tears, the little girl blurted out, "You mean I can never eat anything sweet?" The terror of life without sugar meant a sudden coming to terms with what, for all practical purposes, was a drug addiction to sugar. This girl's ADD was nothing more than the normal bodily response to her sugar addiction.

As a matter of principle, any school system that presumes to offer the best possible learning environment for our children cannot offer them sugar. The soft-drink machine, candy rewards, and bake sales are unhealthy for all and poison for some. Giving children sugar and asking them to learn and behave may be unrealistic.

Attention-Deficit Disorder Caused by Foods

Nine-year-old Trevor appeared with his mother in the office, exhibiting the classic symptoms of attention deficit/hyperactivity disorder. It was not necessary to do a battery of tests to confirm this. (Besides, the furniture and equipment could not have withstood a longer visit.) After discussing the possibility that food intolerance was contributing to Trevor's difficulties at school and at home, we agreed to proceed with the ALCAT Test. Trevor's mother had already noticed that some foods seemed more stimulating to Trevor than others.

Discussing food intolerance with a mother who has thought the problem through and already realizes that some foods are contributing to their child's learning difficulties is a rewarding experience. Within the last year Trevor had begun to have difficulties with grades at school. He had gone from receiving solid A's and B's to getting F's. Teachers had commented to his mother that Trevor was having a hard time concentrating and recommended testing for attention-deficit disorder and Ritalin therapy. Admirably, she resisted this easy way out and began investigating on her own. She learned that foods often contribute to ADD and hyperactivity and was determined to try this avenue before considering drugs for her child.

Trevor was reactive to a number of his favorite foods, including chocolate and cane sugar. Upon learning the results of the ALCAT Test, he exploded in a fit of crying anger when told which foods he would need to eliminate. His mother elegantly accepted the information and started the elimination diet in earnest that day. A week later Trevor and his mom returned. Smiling and relieved, Mom related that Trevor had actually finished all his homework that week and that his grades were much better. He was able to concentrate and his hyperactivity symptoms were much improved. Even Trevor expressed that he felt better and didn't like the feeling he had before.

Surgical Sniffles

A middle-aged surgeon undergoing weight management had chronic rhinitis and sinus drainage. This had caused him considerable discomfort and frequent mask changes during surgery. He was constantly clearing his throat and found it annoying. After having the ALCAT

Test and beginning the elimination diet, his sinus condition and rhinitis cleared up almost immediately. The elimination of reactive foods also allowed him to continue losing weight down to his goal. Months later he continues to maintain his weight by avoiding his reactive foods. His chronic sinus drainage is now only an unpleasant memory.

Foods Can Be a Real Headache

At age 14, John had been suffering classical migraine headaches for several years. The headaches were unpredictable and had ruined a number of family outings for him. Although he avoided the usual foods routinely associated with migraine headaches, he continued to have them unpredictably. Having undergone the usual battery of tests for migraine headache, he was prescribed Imitrex to try and control the headaches after they appeared. The ALCAT Test revealed he was intolerant of a number of foods that neither he nor his family had suspected. Upon his eliminating these foods, John's headaches disappeared. He only experienced a headache when he unintentionally ate a culprit food. After this he became very conscious of avoiding his reactive foods—specifically bananas.

Tired of Fatigue

A 56-year-old grandmother called the doctor's office after the first week of elimination diet proclaiming that her fatigue was gone. After years of debilitating fatigue and gradual weight gain, she felt like a new woman. After a month on the elimination diet based on her ALCAT Test results, her sinus drainage, depression, and burning indigestion had all resolved without medication.

Bad Genes, Yeast, and Food Intolerance

A 40-year-old professional woman and mother of four teenagers came to me for weight management with a chief complaint of "bad genes." Her mother and sisters were all over 20 pounds overweight, and she only dreamed of losing her 20 extra pounds. She had most recently been on a strict 1,000-calorie, low-fat diet and had been exercising vigorously to no avail. Her favorite foods were "sweets and carbohydrates." She admitted eating very fast and had been known to consume entire packages of cookies without remorse.

After discovering her food intolerances via the ALCAT Test, she began her elimination diet with commitment. Her diet was further restricted because of a positive ALCAT Test for *candida* yeast. Using only Nystatin (anti-yeast) as medication, she lost 12 pounds in six weeks. Free of sweet cravings for the first time that she could remember, she now anticipated truly losing to near her ideal weight.

All these people were made sick from the food they ate. Likewise, they became well only after deliberately avoiding the food that caused their illness. If you have food intolerance that is making you ill, only by eliminating that food will you get well. No medication, no surgery, and no therapy will succeed until you eliminate your reactive foods.

To Test or Not to Test

One reason conventional medicine finds it difficult to accept the concept of food sensitivity is that no standard treatment protocol is available. Each patient must be seen and treated on the basis of his or her unique symptoms.

Add to that the time lag of up to 72 hours before symptoms may occur, and the variables boggle the imagination and the office schedule.

Using the interminable method of rotating foods through elimination phases just to detect an improvement in symptoms taxes the perseverance and trust of the most dedicated patient. The ALCAT Test dramatically improves the process of successfully diagnosing and treating food sensitivity reactions. A simple blood test, a few days' wait, and you are ready to climb into the food-elimination saddle. After undergoing the ALCAT Test, you will enter the food elimination phase with a higher degree of confidence and expectation. You will know, with about 80 percent accuracy, the foods to which you are reactive. By yourself or with the help of a knowledgeable practitioner, you can begin eliminating your reactive foods.

It may be wise to seek a professional recommendation as to dietary alternatives and/or specific nutrient supplements, depending on how many and what types of food you need to eliminate. Experience shows that patients notice a significant improvement in various symptoms within the first month; symptoms associated with sinus, headache, and indigestion often improve within two weeks. This is a great impetus to continue the elimination.

Trying to determine my own reactive foods without the benefit of the ALCAT blood test would have been frustrating. Although the test does not pretend to be 100 percent accurate, it eliminates 80 percent of the trial and error that would otherwise be necessary. Just one episode like mine with the chili was enough. The thought of going through that repeatedly during trial-and-error elimination is distasteful (pun intended).

Additionally, the recommended rotation diet that was customized to my own food sensitivities introduced me to a variety of new foods that I still enjoy. Even with hundreds of foods available, most of us eat the same 20 foods in different combinations day after day. All of us would do well to eat a wide variety of fruits and vegetables and decrease the likelihood of developing sensitivities to a particular food that we eat regularly. Without the thorough repertoire of foods allowed and organized for me by the ALCAT Test, eliminating my reactive foods would have been difficult and boring.

Early humans probably did not have to deal with unpleasantries associated with food sensitivity because they, by default, couldn't eat foods not in season or not available to hunt. Today, with a grocery store within a few miles of most Americans, we can indulge in any type of fruit, vegetable, or meat year-round and perpetually stoke the fires of a raging food sensitivity. Science serves us well technologically, but economics prevents the wide dissemination of information that would enable us to make wise choices in our best interest.

We need to know that food sensitivities are a potentially serious problem before we will consider testing to identify and avoid them. Disseminating this preventive information would seem the responsibility of the medical system, yet medical professionals have no great incentive for doing so. After all, if we were to stop getting patients with migraine headaches, ear infections, sinus drainage, indigestion, overweight, coronary artery disease, ADD, hyperactivity, and breathing and skin problems, who will fill the waiting rooms of doctors and hospitals?

CHAPTER 8

Food Sensitivities and Overweight

The likelihood of food sensitivities in individuals who are overweight is strong, if not certain. The very nature of overweight suggests an inappropriate response to food, because it is not uncommon to find overweight people who eat less food and exercise more than might be indicated by their body fat. Rather than insinuate that a person is confused about the volume of food he or she eats, medical professionals should conduct food sensitivity testing to detect any reactive foods. By eliminating these foods, people who test positive for food sensitivities can resume a "normal" weight loss appropriate for calorie intake and exercise.

Let Them Eat Bread

A logical explanation has finally surfaced for the uncontrollable desire to eat inappropriate foods at inappropriate times. Do you crave pasta tonight because of the dinner rolls you ate yesterday? Sound wild? Yes, but wilder yet is the fact that some people who don't eat wheat regularly find themselves getting up in the middle of the night to go buy it. This addiction affliction is like any other. You crave the very substance that is destroying your body. The only differences between food and other addictions are the following:

- Food is legal.
- Food is socially acceptable and encouraged for its known pleasurable pharmacological effects.
- Food addiction/sensitivity produces a variety of symptoms that are treatable on a recurrent basis by your doctor.
- There is no stigma directly associated with food sensitivities (but those suffering from unpredictable bouts of migraine, sinus drainage, eczema, and irritable bowel are stigmatized).

The Heartbreak of Food Sensitivities

The emotional stress placed on those afflicted with food sensitivity is monumental. These individuals may gradually become ostracized by others because of their symptoms, which restrict their activities. This contributes to decreased self-esteem, increased depression, and stress.

These conditions in turn place further demands on the immune system, which is already significantly fatigued by its all-out response to normal foods. To absolve these negative personal feelings, victims often instinctively turn to relief in the form of the chemical serotonin. When present in the brain in adequate amounts, this chemical neurotransmitter can temporarily turn the world rosy. Needless to say, this quick fix fades relatively soon but is easily renewed by the carbohydrate load of a bowl of ice cream, cookies, or pasta (sort of a fix du jour). In fact, those of us conscientious enough to avoid the obviously fat-building foods such as refined sugars can often achieve the same peaceful state by eating (or overeating) pasta, bread, cereal, or any number of refined "low fat" or "no sugar" foods. The dilemma is processed foods that enhance serotonin also stimulate other body hormones such as insulin. The end result is that the more one eats for the serotonin effect, the fatter one gets.

Sadly the serotonin effect is, in the case of food sensitivities, temporary at best. When you eat a food to which you are sensitive, you stress your body, actually creating a decrease in serotonin in the eating center of the brain, but not necessarily immediately. For example, say a person is sensitive to corn. If she eats a food sweetened with corn syrup, or even a corn chip, the immediate result may be a familiar reaction in the body resulting in increased serotonin. Concurrently, however, the food may activate the immune system, resulting in various other chemical reactions depending on the immune system response to the food.

If the cells in the intestinal lining try to control the "invader," one may experience any of various symptoms the body uses to tell us that something is wrong in our intestines. For example, you might experience swelling of the mucosa (lining of the intestine) and a slowing of motility, or constipation, or malabsorption of important nutrients that results in prolific mucous secretion as the irritated lining urges the body to wash this substance away. At this point, the urgent, painful moments on the porcelain throne are legendary.

If the invading food particle is identified and attacked in the blood vessels, this may result in vasculitis, damage to the blood vessel lining. As the blood vessels desperately try to clear this chemical reaction away, they dilate, or open up. This dilation may well lead to severe headaches as well as irritability and muscle pains. Certain foods may cause symptomatic reactions affecting the brain whereas others may affect the sinuses, intestines, skin, or joints. Not every individual will be affected in the same way by each reactive food, but a particular food seems to result in the same symptoms each time it is eaten by the same individual.

Immune Dictatorship

The immune system has total autonomy. If it believes something is bad, our immune system exercises its authority to call forth all the body's energies to protect it. No wonder so many of us with food sensitivities are tired! Once the immune cells have branded a food as an "invader," the food will evoke the wrath of the immune response each time the immune system detects the food in the blood, regardless of how healthy it may seem. And once a food is branded as an invader, each subsequent exposure confirms this. It is a perfect example of "guilty until proven innocent." This results in an incredible amount of resources being wasted fighting an imaginary enemy. As "invader foods" continue to be eaten and absorbed, the body continues consuming body energy, vitamins, and nutrients to maintain the massive "immune army" necessary to keep the body safe from the persistent food invaders.

ALCAT: User Friendly

Ourselves and others who have used the ALCAT food sensitivity test extensively, cannot help but be impressed with its accuracy and versatility. It doesn't simply measure your level of a blood constituent and leave your doctor to figure out what might be causing this abnormality. This form of blood test specifically quantifies the response of your blood to a specific food. The ALCAT test is itself the diagnosis and prescription for treatment—the best of all worlds.

In other words, if you test strongly positive to a food, your treatment is to avoid that food. Cut and dried: simple test, simple treatment. In our day of incredibly complicated tests and interpretations, having a blood test that tells all is a relief.

The ALCAT test is itself the diagnosis and prescription for treatment—the best of all worlds.

To oversimplify the value of this straightforward test would be difficult. Sometimes this raw truth can intimidate patients, who are accustomed to a medical system that often hedges rather than commit to a diagnosis and treatment. Patients are often shocked to find they are reactive to their favorite foods and the recommended treatment is to simply stop eating them. Patients hesitatingly respond, "So if I cut back on eating corn, I will lose weight?"

"No," is the answer. "If you *completely eliminate* all corn and corn products, you can expect all the symptoms relating to eating corn to subside."

After the initial shock has worn off, most are ready to make a rational plan to begin eliminating foods. Depending on the number of reactive foods involved, many patients can begin by eliminating a few of the most frequently eaten foods. After a week or two they should add a few more foods to their elimination list until all are included. However, they must eliminate all reactive foods to confirm whether food intolerance is or is not causing a symptom. Losing weight by spending money on eating the right food is certainly better than spending money on medication.

Feed Me

Food sensitivities may result not only in overeating, but also in malnutrition, by interfering with the metabolism of fat for energy. This results in individuals who are overweight, plagued with "serotonin boosting" cravings, and malnourished because of poor intestinal absorption of nutrients.

Exercise for these patients becomes frustrating when they consume little fat for energy and become hungrier from their exercise. When fat is not accessible to burn for energy, the body falls back on its emergency supply: the small glycogen store in the liver and muscle. Once this readily available source is used up, the body will send you to eat as quickly as possible.

If the biochemical reaction precipitated by food sensitivity blocks your metabolism of fat for energy, you repeatedly tap your emergency carbohydrate supply. Your body then insists you eat to replace this supply, and odds are slim that you will choose pure and natural carbohydrates. You are more likely to consume easily available processed food loaded with sugar and/or fat. At this point, your body is saying, "Feed me. Eat anything, and I will sort it out once it gets here." The result of this hypothetical scenario is that you will have consumed more sugar and fat that will be stored as fat, probably in the form of one or more of your favorite or reactive foods.

This perpetual cycle of living off your emergency supply of carbohydrate results in a slow but steady buildup of fat storage and the feeling of total dependence on carbohydrates for energy. Eventually your brain figures, "The only way out of this cycle is to stop exercising." So let's stop a minute and look at you.

- You have gained weight.
- When you exercise, you don't lose weight but do get hungry.
- You eat right but don't lose weight.
- You stop exercising out of frustration.
- You give in to certain foods that make you feel better.
- You have a food sensitivity!

Fat—How Did This Happen?

Like putting a figurative fence around our fat, the gate only opens into the fat cell; nothing leaves. We must eat, and inevitably, we will eat fat and sugar even as we try to eat healthily. The fat and sugar go to the fat cell through the gate guarded by the chemical response to reactive foods, never to leave again. We can store more fat, but using that fat for energy is prohibited. Imagine being allowed to buy anything you want, but once you take it into your house you can never bring it out again. With time, your only option would be to add to the size of your house. Now your friends bring you things because you have such a large house. Imagine the frustration of people continuing to bring gifts to maintain your large

house when what you want is help taking the furniture
and trash out.

Let's Do Lunch

Overeating as the result of an overwhelming physiologic
response to an allergic chemical reaction occurring somewhere in the body is one thing. Overeating as an inappropriate immediate gratification to emotions such as stress,
anger, or loneliness is another. Actually, when you consider the all-or-nothing laws of nature and physiology, you
might realize that it would be abnormal to not overeat
under certain sets of circumstances. So we manage to:

- Overeat in response to emotions—stress, anger, loneliness, or just out of blatant disregard.

- Repeatedly overuse our favorite foods on a frequent
  "daily" basis, which predisposes us to becoming sensitive
  to these foods.

- Develop chronic symptoms as a result of ongoing chemical reactions precipitated by culprit foods. (These may
  result from repeated overeating of foods, genetically inherited reactions to foods, or pharmacologically mediated reactions to specific chemicals in the foods.)

Somebody Do Something!

Sadly, because of lack of funds for research, we may never
know the exact chemical reactions that lead us to gain and
maintain weight as a response to food sensitivities. To wait

idly for a satisfactory explanation for the impressive results many doctors have noticed is like refusing to tell time until we know how a watch works.

We are not talking about potentially dangerous treatments that require extensive animal and human trials for FDA approval. We are looking at a normal, predictable sequence of events that can be stopped at any time by removing the figurative domino at the start of the chain reaction. After watching this reaction, preventing a repeat would seem straightforward enough—rearrange and remove some dominoes.

Domino Effect

Treating or correcting the infinite maze of reactions created by many foods we eat would seem impossible. In fact, understanding every domino, its angle and tilt, would defy the most intelligent among us. But even you and I can see that if you simply don't tip the first domino, no harm is done. The body's natural response to change is to return to a state of equilibrium. This is what saves us from evolutionarily charging blindly into a brick wall. As the body returns to "normal," the first domino now starts a spontaneous reaction that efficiently proceeds to the more beneficial outcome in the maintenance of life—without sidetracks, split pathways, and dead-ends, and with minimal waste of energy.

Millions of people act as they do and feel as they feel, not by choice, but because their body reacts adversely to a food they have eaten. Much like a parasitic relationship, this chemical response to normal food drains the host's reserves of energy, creates imbalances in brain chemistry, and subverts the host's energy to its purpose. To try to keep up nutritionally with this virtually continuous drain of body energy is like trying to fill a bathtub without plugging the drain.

A Gold Mine of Information

Food sensitivity testing should be and some day will be an integral part of the thorough annual physical examination. Much of the money we currently spend on blood tests is wasted in the sense that we don't get useful information from a normal test. For most blood tests, "normals" are the cumulative averages or most common measurements in a large population sample, which is tantamount to comparing you to everybody else to decide whether you are normal. Doctors order the tests routinely and routinely discount minor abnormalities as "not important" or casually say, "we will check it again next time." If next time is a year later, how valuable was the test in the first place?

Millions of people act as they do and feel as they feel, not by choice, but because their body reacts adversely to a food they have eaten.

In its best-case scenario, an abnormal blood test will lead to more specific tests that either confirm an otherwise undiagnosed condition or confirm that the initial test results were erroneous.

By contrast, consider routine annual testing for food sensitivity. All year long your body fights any number of conditions that cause the absorption of food through a compromised intestinal lining. These conditions may range from pregnancy to viral infection to food poisoning to yeast overgrowth to lack of digestive enzymes. The point is this: Virtually any common everyday condition can result in your body changing its reaction to a particular food.

In the ALCAT test, the "normal" used to standardize the results is your own blood and cells. Thus a normal test is what's normal for you, as opposed to your being compared to a group of strangers.

Doctor, Do Something!

A food that is generally healthy for you can, a week later, set up a cascade of immune and chemical reactions in your body that have far-reaching implications if left undiagnosed. The more frequently you eat this food, the greater the strain on your systems and organs until physical symptoms may take you to your doctor. Baffled by your otherwise good health, your doctor will treat your symptoms as indicated. Unless he or she considers food sensitivities as a possible cause and does appropriate testing, your symptoms are destined to return as you continue eating the culprit food. After an appropriate number of visits, your doctor will add the adjectives "chronic" or "recurrent" in front of your original diagnosis. He or she will do further tests, change your medication, and console you in that you may require continued treatment for this problem for which there is no apparent cure.

Chronic Means "I Don't Know"

You now understand the frustrating plight of the patient with migraine headaches, sinus drainage, ear infections, overweight, irritable bowel syndrome, chronic fatigue, arthritis, and fibromyalgia, to mention a few. All these "conditions" may be merely symptoms of a body's defense system mistaking a normal food for a dangerous invader. It is to your body's credit that this protective mechanism exists and works. Unfortunately, your body uses incredible amounts of energy to protect your immune system and subsequently your organ systems when it is switched on inappropriately.

When your immune system is continuously stressed, protecting you from this food that keeps reappearing, it can no longer maintain its defenses against true invader viruses and bacteria. Likewise, nutrients otherwise destined to support other organ systems are conscripted by the immune system to support its functions. This sets in motion another cascade of events that may eventually result in symptoms of "malnutrition" or deficiencies in nutrients. As each organ system is taxed by the immune system, it may present symptoms that complicate health.

Unless a doctor is insightful enough to consider food sensitivities as the root cause of all your symptoms, your array of diagnoses can be numerous. Each may require medical visits and medication to control symptoms, which in turn leads to low self-esteem. As depression and frustration take over your daily life, you may well become a willing subject of the medical system that seems your only hope.

The nightmare must end. None of this had to happen. Neither you nor your kids had to miss those days of work or school. If food sensitivities were the problem, you didn't have to decline invitations or let your life revolve around medication schedules. Had a relatively painless blood sample been drawn during your annual physical, you would know if you had developed sensitivities to certain foods. Long before the cascade of pathology took place, you could have prevented its progression.

Not only can you treat this problem, but treatment is less expensive than treating a chronic medical condition. Rather than buying medication and keeping doctor appointments for the rest of your life, you simply stop eating your reactive food or foods for a period of time. Often after three to six months, you can begin reintroducing these foods into your diet if you wish. All in all, you save instead of spend money to cure this condition. You stop buying your reactive foods, you add new foods to your diet, and you learn the most basic of lessons: Your health is your responsibility. No one knows your body better than you do. Unless you actively *lead* those caring for your health, you *follow* them.

This brings us back to my original contention, that food sensitivity testing is more valuable than most screening tests done today. Even a negative or "normal" test reinforces your eating habits and skills and allows you to safely assume that any symptoms you develop are not food related. Once we realize the tremendous potential food has to enrich as well as to unravel our lives, we stop taking it for granted.

The Politics of Food Sensitivities

As Scott Peck, M.D., so simply yet eloquently states in the first chapter of his 1986 book *The Road Less Traveled:* "Life is difficult." He goes on to discuss that once it is accepted that life is difficult, "the fact that life is difficult no longer matters. . . . What makes life difficult is that the process of confronting and solving problems is a painful one, yet it is in this whole process of meeting and solving problems, that life has meaning." Dr. Peck puts in perspective life and the choices we make.

Those who only accept life as purely scientifically justified have long relegated the treatment of overweight to the shadows of medicine. These same individuals can offer no scientifically justified and confirmed treatment for overweight. In lieu of this, they willingly continue to treat patients' symptoms with stopgap medications. These patients are then criticized for trying to control overweight through alternative methods by the same people who offer no reliable medical treatment for their disease—an apparent "catch-22" situation. The art and the business of medicine seem to be in great conflict with regard to treating overweight. Life *is* difficult.

Food sensitivities/allergies have been a confirmed cause of human illness since the beginning of this century when Hamburger and Schloss confirmed the first known cases of food allergies. In that time frame, conventional medicine has accepted, denied, partially accepted, and totally denigrated food sensitivity as a true condition. This seemingly confused approach to food allergies stems from a number of issues:

- **Political.** To accept food as a cause of illness would contradict many influential scientists and divert funds from their research into curing disease with medication.
- **Medical philosophy.** Current medical doctrine is based on nonfood causes of disease. For example, the symptoms of a child's cold can be traced to the release of chemicals by the immune system, resulting in the release of protective body reactions to isolate and eliminate the offending agent. It is obvious (or it's too difficult to consider other causes) that an organism

is the cause of a cold because of the way our immune
system reacts. In the era of HMOs and big business medicine, the common accepted treatment is the one that
will be paid for. There is little incentive for an individual
practitioner to consider patients as individuals whose
common symptoms may be unrelated to the conventional "odds."

- **The wide array of symptoms caused by food allergies.**
  The varying symptoms related to food sensitivity per-
  plexes the practitioner who is under pressure to give relief now. Americans are not given to dealing with
  problems for the long term; we are addicted to instant
  gratification. Our medical system struggles to live up to
  our expectations and still remain highly profitable. This
  precludes recommending an elimination diet that ex-
  cludes what are likely your favorite foods. Because the
  best-case scenario—that your condition resolves and you
  don't need to see your doctor again—is hardly a prac-
  tice-building activity, your caregiver will more likely supply the conventional medication and recommend you
  return if the condition doesn't improve.

- **The lack of concrete evidence as to the exact mechanisms by which food allergies perpetuate their symptoms.** This is the clincher for many physicians who need
  the full faith and confidence of their medical textbooks
  and literature behind each treatment. In all fairness,
  our medical/legal atmosphere perpetuates the "conventional" practice. Few physicians continue to learn with
  each patient they treat. Learning comes via the drug
  and medical equipment companies that sponsor continuing education or visit offices to update doctors on
  newer drugs. Drug companies seldom encourage doctors to consider something as mundane as food as the
  cause of and cure for patients' health problems. If you
  cure your migraine with food elimination, who will buy

the headache medicine? If your irritable bowel settles when you stop eating a food, who will finance the x-ray department at the hospital?

So as you can see, the medical establishment has little incentive to promote research into food allergies. Even if research identified the cause of food allergies, you can be sure that, unless big drug companies make a pill to alleviate your symptoms, it will not be highly touted.

Without having a complete understanding of how a clock works, one can predictably and reliably know the time of day. Likewise, treating food allergies is a science of noticing the symptoms, then not noticing them once foods are eliminated. In efforts to help patients, doctors don't have to agree with all the intricate details of how food allergies cause illness, but need only be aware that food allergies may explain their symptoms.

Do No Harm

There is no question that caution is a virtue in conventional medicine. When doctors treat a patient with a prescription medication, they must concede they usually don't know how the medication works at the cellular level. Therefore, they depend on careful and thorough testing by the drug company before using the medication for patients. But this slow, time-consuming evaluation seems overkill when applied to a therapeutic mechanism that removes a food from the diet. Asking patients to eliminate some foods to see whether they get relief is hard enough for doctors, but realizing that patients can cure themselves without the prescription pad is humbling.

Even those who are closed-minded regarding food sensitivity testing realize that some foods are more allergy provoking than others. This awareness may enable these doctors to successfully treat many patients with food intolerance without drugs, or to relegate patient care to nutritionists, osteopaths, homeopaths, and dietitians familiar with advances in food sensitivity testing for food allergies.

Doctors for the most part do have intense concern for their patients. Sooner or later their compassion will lead them to consider the growing body of evidence that our food may be making us sick. The long-term health benefits of proper eating are undeniable, and to eat properly you must know the foods to which your body will react abnormally. Avoiding these allergic reactions is imperative to maintaining your good health.

Synopsis

1. Food is legal and can be selectively used for its pleasant pharmacological effects.
2. Recurring use of foods may result in recurring symptoms from sensitivities and result in recurring medical visits.
3. Food sensitivities/addictions may be legal, but the psychological distress of the resulting obesity and the many related physical maladies are socially more confining than a physical jail.
4. There is a sound physiologic basis for the signs and symptoms associated with food sensitivities.
5. ALCAT food sensitivity testing is a consistently accurate, cost-effective method of food sensitivity testing.
6. Eliminating foods to which you are reactive resolves symptoms caused by food allergies.
7. Conventional medicine condones the use of medications with confirmed adverse side effects as long as the side effects are known and documented.

8. Elimination of a food to which you are reactive has no adverse side effects.

9. Politics, economics, and medical bureaucracy may have conflicts of interest in advocating the elimination of food sensitivities to treat disease.

CHAPTER 9

The Right Diet for the 21st Century

For years, various doctors and other health care professionals have noticed that patients who removed allergenic foods from their diets for any reason experienced a welcome side effect: They lost weight. Now, two breakthrough research studies have shown that this side effect is not just coincidental—they conclusively establish that eating allergenic foods contributes to weight gain in a large percentage of the population. How this occurs is not exactly understood, but research and practical experience suggest that three mechanisms are involved: the brain chemicals that trigger food addiction, the body's individual rate of metabolism, and the damage to blood vessels that causes edema.

A main reason traditional weight loss diets often do not work is that they do not eliminate foods that an overweight cannot tolerate. The allergenic food then triggers one or more reactions, which locks the overweight person in a merciless cycle of weight gain. Any foods (and often the very foods that are craved most) can cause these problems.

Food Allergies Finally Getting Some Respect

Over the last five years there has been a steady increased interest and attention to food allergies and their contribution to many medical conditions. Rarely does a week go by that there is not some reference to food allergies in the popular press. Psychologists and psychiatrists now use elimination of food allergies to treat depression's underlying cause even when they may use antidepressants short term. Repairing the brain chemistry is much better than taking medications forever. One national alcohol treatment program uses food allergy testing to determine grains and particular foods that may specifically be related to the depression and anxiety that leads to drinking. Fibromyalgia treatment centers and physicians use food allergy testing to precisely identify foods that may be causing fibromyalgia.

Conventional medicine is slow to accept change. But open-minded intellectuals are always trying to find better ways to help others. Contrary to common opinion, we haven't discovered everything there is to know about the human body yet. For those individuals who find themselves falling through the cracks of conventional medical treatment the option of treating their disease without another medication is a welcome one.

The call for alternative therapies has also invoked attention to food allergy testing and elimination. People are just tired of paying the outrageous prices for medicine that they are going to have to take forever unless they figure out what the underlying cause of their problem is. It is as though conventional HMO medicine were "Band-Aid" medicine. Cover it up and move on to the next one. To get the help they need people are learning to search out the doctors who are slow to recommend prescription chemicals, and are more interested in running down the cause of a problem than covering it up.

Good News for Food Addicts

The good news is that when overweight people remove intolerant foods from their diet, their brain chemicals, metabolism, and digestive system normalize. Their food addictions vanish, their metabolism functions at its optimum rate, and their water retention disappears—all without the deprivation of low-calorie diets, without dangerous diet drugs, and without endless hours of exercise. What's more, groundbreaking studies on food intolerance and weight loss conducted using the ALCAT test show that when people cut their intolerant foods from their diets, they lose not just weight, but fat, and in many cases gain lean muscle. It bears stating again here that any realistic healthy diet plan will be maximally enhanced by avoiding one's reactive foods. For those who need accountability or who feel they must pay for special food supplements to lose weight, the good news is that by knowing your food allergies and avoiding them, you can make even an expensive weight loss program work better.

Kaats Research

Controlling body fat is as simple as controlling food allergies. That was the conclusion of groundbreaking research conducted in 1995 by Gilbert Kaats, Ph.D., director of the Health and Medical Research Foundation in San Antonio, Texas.

Thirty patients on a low-caloric diet plateaued in terms of weight loss. In a sequential phase of the same study, they continued low-caloric diets but also eliminated ALCAT-positive foods. Weight loss resumed, and before-and-after determinations of body composition showed that their weight loss was fat. Most interestingly, women lost fat from the hips. What you eat is more important than how much you eat. This concept overturns the commonly held belief that food quantity is the culprit in overweight, a belief that is clearly not correct.

Addictive Overeating and Food Intolerance

The findings of these two important studies correlate with many other current studies on the relationship among individual biochemistry, food addiction, and body weight and health. Changing attitudes and new research on obesity is leading to increased interest in just what triggers overeating behavior and drives people to eat their way into obesity.

For years, psychiatrists and psychologists have observed food addiction patterns where patients have a constant craving for food (especially candy, ice cream, and other sweets) that compels them to eat far beyond their energy requirements. They crave food like an alcoholic craves a drink or a smoker a cigarette. Doctors and weight loss specialists have been frustrated in their efforts to help these people lose weight. Many practitioners now believe that these irresistible cravings may stem from a biochemical dependency that can sabotage any weight control program. Allergenic foods may drive you to overeat instead of break out in a rash.

It has been suggested that obesity is associated with a defect in the appetite control system. Science is now showing us conclusively that certain foods and food chemicals trigger changes in brain chemistry that result in allergy-like, addictive overeating. Dr. F. Fuller Royal, a clinical ecologist and modern pioneer in the field of food sensitivities and environmental medicine, wrote, "I have come to realize that a very high percentage (80 percent) of obese patients have serious food allergy-addiction. They will never be able to adequately conquer the problems of obesity . . . until their allergic-addictive foods have been identified and eliminated from their diets." The only problem with this solution, until recently, has been identifying the offending foods. Before the ALCAT test, this was a difficult, expensive, and time-consuming process.

Doctors' Experiences

Doctors who use the simple ALCAT blood test have conquered the difficulties in identifying food sensitivities and are reporting such unprecedented results in helping patients control weight as the following:

> As soon as I started avoiding the foods I tested sensitive to, I began losing one to one-and-a-half pounds a week without changing my activity level or consciously reducing portions. I found I wasn't as hungry and had fewer cravings, so it was the easiest and most successful diet I've ever been on.
>
> —Dr. John Magauran, general practitioner,
> Honolulu, Hawaii

> I tell my patients it makes sense to know your food hypersensitivities. Some of my greatest successes are members of the Austrian Ski Team, who went on to win Olympic medals.
>
> —Dr. Stephen Schimpf, preventive medicine
> and immunotherapy, Salzburg, Austria

> We tested people who had stopped losing weight. Once we eliminated their sensitive foods they lost fat and kept it off.
>
> —Dr. Richard Bahr, environmental medicine,
> Cincinnati, Ohio

> Patients who attempt to lose weight and keep it off aren't successful until they eliminate their allergenic foods.
>
> —Dr. Barbara Solomon, internal medicine,
> Baltimore, Maryland

One of the positive side effects of the ALCAT program for many of my patients is that they also lose weight.

—Dr. Stephen Smith, allergy and skin,
Richland, Washington

Until I started using the ALCAT test, I was missing some foods, chemicals, and preservatives with my patients. Now I use it as the main instrument for testing for food allergies in a variety of conditions including weight loss, and when I can't diagnose anything definite.

—Dr. Paul Jaconello, nutrition and preventive medicine,
Toronto, Ontario

We have found the ALCAT testing and the elimination diet to be a useful tool as a part of a program to lose weight and maintain weight loss.

—Dr. James F. Bain, family practice,
director of Wabash Physician Services

In my judgment, the ALCAT test has been very useful in diagnosing food sensitivities. One of the most interesting cases is that of a young girl with eosinophilic gastroenteritis. Management of this patient was difficult until use of the ALCAT test identified her problem foods. I have also observed that a great many of my food-sensitive patients lose weight as a result of following the exclusionary diet prescribed by the test and that this is due to something other than restriction of calorie intake.

—Dr. Leland Green, board-certified allergist,
Lansdale, Pennsylvania

I have never found anything better for diagnosing food sensitivities in children than the ALCAT test. I have used it extensively for many years and have found it to be especially helpful with the more complicated cases. It is also very useful for identifying adverse reactions to the food additives, chemicals, and antibiotics. The potential effects of these substances are a very important consideration.

—Dr. Walter Ward, ENT allergy and environmental medicine,
Winston-Salem, North Carolina

Beyond the Zone

One interesting note comes from Barry Sears through his popular book *The Zone,* in which he discusses the important relationship of hormones to obesity. His complex theory revolves around certain superhormones called eicosanoids. Actually, eicosanoids are not technically hormones but autacoids, because they exert their effect locally in the tissue in which they are formed rather than systemically as circulating hormones. This particular aspect of eicosanoids makes their application to food intolerance that much more understandable. One perplexing aspect of food intolerance has been its seemingly inconsistent presentation of symptoms in a variety of organ systems. This is now clarified by understanding that tissues have different eicosanoid-binding sites. That is, certain eicosanoids affect certain tissues preferentially. Depending on the particular eicosanoid reaction to food intolerance, symptoms may appear as gastrointestinal, respiratory, vascular, or dermatological. For that matter, any organ system may be affected.

Certain eicosanoids are produced in adipose tissue and are potent regulators of the breakdown of fat. In particular, PGE-2 (prostaglandin E-2) inhibits lipolysis. That means it prevents the breakdown of fat for energy. Anything that increases the synthesis of this eicosanoid may prevent you from using your own fat stores for energy, regardless of how much you exercise. Add to this the antilipolytic (inhibits lipolysis) effect of insulin, and you may become a carbohydrate junkie to meet your basic metabolic energy requirements. Also synthesized by adipose tissue is PGI-2. This eicosanoid promotes the breakdown of fat and is lipolytic in its action. The coordinated modulation of these two eicosanoids results in what most of us consider normal fat metabolism. But when one eicosanoid is synthesized preferentially over the other, an imbalance of fat metabolism occurs.

Who Are Those Guys?

Eicosanoids are arachidonic acid metabolites. Arachidonic acid is an essential fatty acid that must be supplied in the diet, as the body has no way of deriving it from normal metabolic pathways. Arachidonic acid exists in the plasma membrane of all cells. Eicosanoid synthesis depends on a variety of chemically and hormonally mediated events. The particular eicosanoids synthesized in a tissue are determined by the enzyme systems present in that tissue. Thus some eicosanoids may affect many cells, albeit in different ways. Others may exert their effect in only a few select tissues.

What Does This Have to Do with Food?

Food intolerance results in an inflammatory reaction mediated by the immune system. Inflammation results in or from the synthesis of eicosanoids. For example, the polymorphonuclear white blood cells (also known as granulocytes because they contain granules of destructive chemicals) that engulf and destroy allergenic food particles (a process also known as phagocytosis) release PGE-2. Furthermore, PGE-2 depresses lymphocyte function and may result in depressed cellular immunity. PGE-2 also causes vasodilation and increased vascular permeability. This results in local tissue edema and fluid retention. PGE-2 has known adverse effects on fat metabolism, blood vessel permeability, insulin production, gastric acid output, platelet aggregation, and bronchoconstriction and can result in immune system suppression, dysmenorrhea, and inflammation. If all this can come from a reaction to a food, we are far beyond worrying whether eating ice cream would ruin our diet.

Why Hasn't Anyone Told Me?

Throughout this book we have stressed the need for further research into the relationship of food intolerance and chronic disease. Before such research is concluded, thousands of eicosanoids may be identified. The example of PGE-2 used here may be only a start. Even today many eicosanoids are recognized whose function and activity are uncertain. The question is, Do you want to learn how to make a watch, or do you want to know what time it is?

The point is that for now it is only interesting to know the postulated mechanism by which food intolerance may affect overweight and other chronic conditions. Forget about how it happens; just realize it is happening. Realize that you control the reactions that take place in your body by the foods you choose to eat.

How Does It Work?

What we take for granted as a "normal" diet is a relatively recent cultural development. For one thing, until recently people in many parts of the world were never exposed to foods not indigenous to their area. In some instances, the modern diet has outstripped biological mechanisms of adaptation. As was previously mentioned, members of certain population groups have not evolved the digestive enzymes needed to fully digest cow's milk protein, a relatively recent evolutionary event. According to *Harrison's Principles of Internal Medicine*, 13th edition, 1994, about 5 to 15 percent of the adult white population shows intestinal lactase deficiency, but African-Americans and Asians are about 80 to 90 percent lactose intolerant.

In the last 50 years our diet has changed dramatically. The same digestive enzymes that were needed to digest only fresh fruits and vegetables and range-fed meats must now somehow deal with the huge amounts of preservatives, colorings, chemical fertilizers, insecticides, and antibiotics in our foods. As our digestive enzymes fall short, our immune systems react to these substances to protect us from the toxic consequences.

Food intolerance knocks the body's biochemistry out of balance. As a result, the metabolism becomes sluggish, the immune system becomes impaired, the digestive tract develops leaks, insulin and other hormones become imbalanced, and the body loses control of the neurotransmitters that control appetite. Your brain assimilates all this and sends the message "You are falling apart."

Alterations of the chemicals that control appetite trigger food cravings and eating binges; disruption of normal metabolism impacts how much fat is stored; and damage to the vascular system causes fluid to leak into connective tissues, which results in water retention. All in all, not a pretty picture. But there's hope. Research studies using the ALCAT test have shown, as has the Kaats study performed at Baylor, that once you take care of your food intolerances, your body is able to lose fat. Also, Dr. Cabo-Soler, Professor of Biochemistry at the University of Valencia of Spain, found, in 1998, that dieters who had plateaued on a low calorie diet lost more fat, and women especially lost fat from their hip region, by just avoiding the foods indicated by the ALCAT test, with no further calorie restriction or exercise.

It's suspected that by removing the food disruptions, the body's mechanisms normalize, reducing the body's physiological craving for sweets and carbohydrates, normalizing the body's hunger mechanisms, and returning to efficient fat burning. What's more, with these food disturbances out of your system, you will feel healthier and more energetic. This increases the chance that you will exercise.

No One-Size-Fits-All Diet Exists

Overweight people share one common denominator—they have too much stored fat tissue. Their paths to overweight may be as randomly different as the patterns formed by snowflakes. And yet many cookie-cutter diets are touted. Who's looking out for the individual? Few recognize the powerful mechanisms that make each person unique—for example, inherited difference of hormones and metabolism, environmental variations in exposure to pollution, lifestyle differences of stress, and particular food choices affecting the individual. The key is to understand and adapt the diet to the powerful forces that help to determine body weight.

Following a weight loss diet that instructs you to eat one orange, an egg, and toast for breakfast may sound healthy and well balanced. But what if you're intolerant to eggs? What if that very egg you ate caused your blood cells to expand and explode, and this reaction caused your serotonin level to plummet and send a message from your brain to eat more carbohydrate? You're going to find it hard to lose weight on that diet. The problem seems to arise from the fact that some foods have been declared universally healthy by popular acclaim. There are no universally safe foods, with the possible exception of pure water.

Because you are not a clone of your neighbor, you need a diet that takes your uniqueness into consideration. If you're intolerant to tuna, you don't have tuna sandwiches for lunch no matter what your friend eats. Clothes look different on your body, perfumes smell different on your skin, and food acts different inside. *Vive la différence!*

There are no universally safe foods, with the possible exception of pure water.

If we truly intend to treat obesity as the medical problem it is claimed to be, how can one dietary solution work for every person? Other medical problems do not have a single solution. When treating other diseases and conditions, doctors take into account each patient's medical history, degree of illness, reaction to pharmaceuticals, and other information. Then they design a treatment plan for that person. Weight loss deserves the same one-on-one attention, because no two people are genetically, biochemically, or psychologically the same.

Obesity is recognized as a chronic medical condition because of its impact on other organ systems and overall health. Its solution, however, may lie in the use of less medication. Identifying reactive foods and avoiding them may represent the indicated medical treatment for this "plague." So many subtle functions within the cells defend the body from the effects of the minute but powerful eicosanoids. These trigger waves of hormonal activity, and the expulsion of powerful mediating chemicals, which go about eliminating or neutralizing invaders like law enforcement officers with stun guns at a riot.

Now we have a scientifically proven method for identifying offending foods and food substances that can be applied to a broad range of programs and have a profound effect in reducing health care costs.

Drugs, the Dieter's Tow Truck

Drugs are for the most part very effective clinically, but they work from outside the body's basic chemistry to affect only hunger or cravings. Once they wear off, the underlying biochemistry returns to its previous hungry, craving mode. Drugs have a number of drawbacks in terms of side effects, cost, and the need for long-term use to artificially modulate hunger and cravings. They fail to keep weight off long term if food intolerances are not identified and eliminated.

Of even greater concern is the relatively poor track record of appetite suppressant drugs in recent years. Many have been discovered to be dangerous to large segments of the population. Nevertheless, paying little attention, Americans clamor for their prescriptions and take the medications. Because they don't correct any deficiencies or biochemical aberrations, appetite suppressants are like a metabolic tow truck. Just as when your car is broken down, the tow truck is a welcome sight to get you to where repairs are available. None of us would decline repairs to our car and pay the tow truck to keep towing us everywhere. Likewise, appetite suppressants are valuable in the limited context that they are medications with side effects and are expensive. The realistic use of appetite suppressant medications is for short-term use, to allow us to diagnose and fix the problem. So rather than to expect doctors and their medications to tow you around the rest of their lives, insist that they do the tests: thyroid, candida yeast, and ALCAT. Through the use of these tests, many of the underlying causes of overweight can be discovered and treated effectively while short-term drugs tide you over.

Candida yeast overgrowth may also be a factor in weight gain. In particular, because it causes the body to crave sugar, which feeds the candida yeast organisms, causing them to grow. Sugar also increases production of insulin, which pushes the sugar out of the bloodstream and deposits it, as fat, into the fat cells. Muscle metabolism only allows sugar into the cells very slowly; the body will not tolerate extended periods of high sugar levels in the blood. In the effort to control these high sugar levels the body will quite rapidly dispose of the sugar by converting it and storing it safely away as fat. Therefore, candida overgrowth, as well as anything else that increases sugar cravings (or, cravings of foods with a high glycemic index) such as food intolerance, will, if the cravings are satisfied, lead to increase in fat tissue.

Intestinal yeast overgrowth is a known risk factor in the development of food intolerance. As mentioned elsewhere, yeast overgrowth in the gut is thought to contribute to the condition called "leaky gut." The term alludes to the leaking of intestinal contents consisting of digested and undigested food through the normally exquisitely effective intestinal lining filter. This results in inordinately large particles of undigested food entering the bloodstream. At this point the body proceeds to complete digestion of the food but fingerprints it as a foreign invader. When the specialized cells in the bloodstream see this food particle again in the future, more immune system cells are called forward each time.

Eventually, full-blown symptoms of allergy result as the body becomes convinced that it is being invaded and does all it can to expel the invader by causing inflammation to limit its spread. Treating the yeast without considering the possibility of food intolerance is only partially treating a person's overweight problem. Every patient I have tested for food sensitivities and who also had confirmed tests for excessive candida yeast overgrowth has had an extensive list of food sensitivities.

And to piece this puzzle together even further, in 1977 a study on yeast was done and reported in the *Journal of the American Medical Association (JAMA)*. Miles and his associates found a direct correlation between vaginal yeast and simultaneous overgrowth of candida in the intestinal tract. If you are a woman who has been plagued with recurrent vaginal yeast infections or even if you only suffer yeast infections when you take antibiotics, you seem likely to have food sensitivities. If overweight, sinus congestion, reflux, headaches, fatigue, asthma, or unusually strong cravings for sweets are an issue for you, get tested for food sensitivities.

Low-calorie diets work initially, if a person has unidentified food intolerances but weight regain is all too often speedier than the weight loss was. The biochemical aberrations produced as a result of food reactions will overpower any willpower. It is as though the food sensitivity had you chained to the refrigerator door.

Intense aerobic exercise should control excess fat but often fails to meet expectations if a person has unidentified food intolerance. Exercise alone has rarely been successful in eliminating excess body fat. It must be accompanied by dietary adjustments, and it is impossible to know which foods to eat until you know your food intolerances.

So you see, although other aspects of controlling and maintaining weight may all have a place, knowing your food limitations is the secret to controlling your overweight. Everyone needs to exercise in some fashion, even if that just means moving around more. Diet drugs may be useful in defraying the urges to overeat while you focus on eliminating foods that cause cravings. Reasonable calorie control is obviously necessary to prevent weight gain. And control of candidiasis is useful in alleviating some sweet cravings and correcting intestinal function. But food intolerance and the subtle effects it has on eicosanoids, insulin, the thyroid, serotonin, the immune system, nutrient absorption, and digestion are a whole different dimension from overeating food because it looks or tastes good.

What makes any program work better, what holds it all together, is knowing and understanding your food intolerances.

One Simple Blood Test

Unfortunately, we may never know the exact chemical reactions that lead to weight gain and maintenance of overweight as a result of food intolerance because we lack funds for research. But to wait idly for a satisfactory explanation for the impressive results would deny millions the potential for improving their lives.

The ALCAT test has a great track record. Many studies and reports substantiate it as the premier test to determine foods to which the individual is intolerant. A state-of-the-art evolution of blood tests that evaluate the individual's cellular response to an allergic substance, the test consists of making measurements of white blood cells and platelets in an individual's blood specimen. The whole blood is then exposed to common food extracts and chemicals. The specific reaction of the cells to these foods and chemicals then tells the story. Changes occur in these blood cells if they have been programmed by the body to react to the food and chemicals in question. By detecting and quantifying the degree of change in the blood cells, the ALCAT test then determines the degree of reactivity the tested individual has to the substance.

Because each determination is calibrated to the individual's own blood, there is no "normal" to look up in a book. In other words, a normal response is the response of the same individual's blood before the food or chemical is introduced. The ALCAT test's highly individualized nature makes it preferable over tests that report results in the broad "normal" range for the general population. Confirmation comes through the relief of symptoms as one eliminates the culprit foods from the diet. The simplicity of the concept belies how intricate the actual process is. This is pure medicine, in that curing the disease rather than covering it up relieves symptoms.

We are not talking potentially dangerous treatments or drugs that require extensive trials and studies to confirm their safety. We are talking common sense that confounds the tenets of scientific investigation. After all, what is common sense to one is heresy to another. But while the purists study, and while the drug companies seek further ways to profit, you and I can heal ourselves by understanding that food may be causing many of our miseries and by avoiding the foods that do.

Piecing the Puzzle Together

As we cruise into the 21st century, we have to reverse the terrible trends associated with obesity. This can be done in the conventional way by treating each symptom as it appears or it can be done the ALCAT way—accepting food intolerance as a real disease and treating the cause to reduce the incidence of symptoms: obesity, ADD, migraines, irritable bowel syndrome, colitis, depression, reflux gastritis, arthritis, and sinusitis, among others. During most of the 20th century, these were considered diseases that had no real cure and could only be treated symptomatically. Medical experts now know that in many cases they were only symptoms of the underlying condition of food intolerance.

This century will find us using selective food elimination and consumption to improve the quality of our lives. Simple blood tests such as the ALCAT test will guide us through the maze of available foods.

But don't wait! Start now to use food as your medicine. If you are now trying to lose weight or contemplating starting a weight loss program, learn what foods you do not tolerate. Supercharge any sensible weight loss program and make it last by understanding food intolerance and its cure. Lose weight by applying yourself diligently to limiting unnecessary calories, taking in plenty of nutrients, and avoiding foods to which you react badly. Finally, a practical solution: Avoid your untolerated foods, and cravings will disappear, leaving you to concentrate on eating foods that will supply nutrients. Energy levels will improve, and exercise will become a realistic option. Think clearly, run faster, and love living.

The new hunter-gatherer searches in earnest for nutrient to maximize his or her potential and shuns food that limits his or her mental and physical well-being: "Thou shalt not eat of the forbidden fruit." And the forbidden fruit is determined by your body's reaction to foods you choose. Know your forbidden foods, and avoid them.

Nutrient-Driven Eating

One outstanding feature of the ALCAT test is that, along with identifying your food reactivities, it reports your safe foods as well. This means you not only have a good idea which foods may be making you sick, but also have a ready selection to use in lieu of your reactive foods. This is especially important for cases in which the food to be eliminated represents a substantial source of a particular vitamin or mineral. For example, if you found you were reactive to carrots, and they were your only significant source of beta-carotene, eliminating them could result in a serious deficiency of vitamin A in your body. Supplements can cover this shortage until you are able to resume eating your untolerated foods, usually after about 90 days.

However, with guidance you will be able to identify several other rich sources of beta-carotene among the list of "safe" foods in the ALCAT report manual. Minerals likewise must be accounted for if rich sources are eliminated. For example, if you eliminate milk, taking calcium supplements or choosing to eat calcium-rich "safe" foods would be wise.

Although most of us feel uncomfortable with the responsibility of replacing deficient vitamins and minerals in our bodies, we shouldn't. That is what eating is. The fact that we willingly delegate our nutritional replenishment to the short-order cook at the fast-food restaurant is the epitome of irresponsibility. To regain control of our health, we must reclaim responsibility for what we eat. Hidden food allergies begin all too often as a result of mindless eating of nutrient-depleted processed foods on a daily basis. We often eat only our favorite foods, eat too fast, and eat for reasons other than hunger.

Rotate, Rotate, Rotate

Blind luck would give us better nutrition if we varied our food choices from day to day. The rotation diet concept has long been a standard for avoiding the development of food intolerance. As a general rule, avoid eating a food more often than every fourth day, and your chances of developing food intolerance diminish. In our fast food-dependent society, this takes more planning than just eating at a different restaurant each day. We must give especially careful thought to avoiding foods such as wheat, corn, milk, soy, and eggs, because they appear in so many different forms of fast food. As a matter of fact, eating out becomes a greater hassle than it is worth as we attempt to avoid foods we know are bad for us. As an aid, the ALCAT test results report includes a four-day planned rotation diet of the theoretically "safe foods."

"But I Take a Multivitamin"

A healthy body is the result of careful planning. On our behalf, the Food and Drug Administration has calculated the amounts of various vitamins and minerals necessary to prevent deficiency states. The recommended amounts necessary to keep from showing signs of deficiency are reported as RDAs, or recommended daily allowances, as standards for food labeling. To me, the thought of taking just enough vitamin C to keep scurvy away seems a bit passive.

Recently, the *University Wellness Letter,* a well-known health reference, has recommended vitamin C doses of 500 mg per day and vitamin E of 400 to 800 mg per day. This represents a shift away from minimum doses to prevent signs of deficiency and a groundswell toward doses of vitamins and nutrients to therapeutically promote health. More important, this suggests some useful research may be forthcoming regarding using nutrients to prevent disease.

First of all, the human body gets its most usable form of nutrients, vitamins, and minerals from fruits, seeds, nuts, vegetables, unprocessed grains, meat, and fish. Other sources are less usable by the body. Artificial supplements should not be taken in lieu of eating properly but to enhance the body's ability to fight disease. Taking vitamins to substitute for eating carefully is like substituting a Ford Pinto for a limousine. It may get you there, but it just won't be the same, and you won't feel nearly as good.

So don't choke down the once-a-day vitamin and think you have done your duty. Your intestine likely will treat it like the armored nugget it is and may chip the porcelain off the toilet bowl. Take your vitamin and mineral supplements at various times during the day and be sure they are likely to dissolve in your gut. (Your pills should dissolve in 30 minutes in vinegar if they are likely to do you any good at all!) The intestine is designed to absorb a steady stream of nutrients all day, so present your supplements in this way.

Feeding the Immune System

As one recovers from the often devastating effects of food intolerance, recognizing and correcting deficiencies that have developed in the body is also important. Eliminating the culprit foods gives the immune system some respite, some breathing room, if you will. The problem is that to some extent the damage has been done.

The various immune cells have been overworked for some time. This has set in place the natural cascade of reactions that follows depletion of immune cell nutrients. This sequence of reactions can result in misfiring of the immune system cells. Because the network of cells making up your immune system depends on continuous communication, failure of any part of your system may result in a rogue immune system that may attack your body itself. This autoimmune destruction of body tissues is classic in many chronic diseases. Rather than selectively treating these autoimmune diseases, you would do well to initiate nutritional resuscitation of the immune system so as to minimize permanent damage to your body tissues. Even before your food intolerance is completely resolved, it is important that you begin rehabilitating your weakened immune system. Assuming poor absorption from the intestinal tract, supplementing vitamins and minerals vital to assure healthy immune system functioning is warranted. These supplements, combined with an appropriate elimination diet, will begin to normalize the digestion, absorption, and metabolism of nutrients needed to correct conditions brought about by immune system attacks on the body itself. Keep in mind that the malnourished and overactive immune system leads to many symptoms of food intolerance.

Some well-established immune system nutrients and suggested supplemental dosages are as follows:

Vitamin E. 400-800 mg/day is generally accepted as safe. This powerful antioxidant is a confirmed immune system potentiator. Use mixed tocopherols to include gamma-tocopherol. If choices are limited, avoid DL tocopherol.

Vitamin C. 1,000 mg/day in divided doses is conservative, and up to 10,000 mg/day may be justified in times of illness, because the body consumes enormous amounts under stress. Every immune system function benefits from the presence of vitamin C. Loose bowels is an upper limit sign, and the dose should be decreased until loose bowel movements resolve.

Beta-carotene. 15 mg/day or 25,000 units/day are recommended. This precursor to vitamin A is a highly regarded immune system stimulant. Several studies have documented its benefits in cancer prevention, and it is necessary for some immune cells to mature properly.

Selenium 100–200 mg/day. This potent antioxidant teams up with vitamin E to protect cells.

B vitamins. This group of vitamins is best taken in a "complex" containing the range of B vitamins. Vitamin B_6 is especially susceptible to deficiency from poor absorption. University studies confirm that vitamin B_6 plays an important role in the immune system. Stress results in B vitamin wasting, and deficiency in virtually any of the B vitamins may lead to depression. Vitamins B_6 and B_{12} are necessary to prevent homocystine, a potent predictor of heart disease. Deficiency of folic acid has been linked to birth defects.

Zinc. 30 mg/day of this mineral is invaluable for immune cell development and activity. Immune system activity consumes large quantities of zinc. Zinc supplements should be taken separate from multivitamin supplements, because copper and iron may inhibit the absorption of zinc. Take zinc at supper to enhance healthy production of insulin as you sleep.

Calcium. 1,000 mg/day. This mineral is necessary for the activation of complement, a component of the immune system that works with antibodies to destroy bacteria.

Magnesium. 500 mg/day is recommended. Deficiency depresses immunoglobulins needed to fight bacterial and viral infection. Many amino acid functions and biochemical reactions are magnesium dependent. Magnesium is also needed to facilitate the strengthening of bone. Magnesium is a natural sedative and enhances bowel function.

Copper. 3 mg/day. The exact role of copper is not known, but deficiency leads to suppressed immune function.

Iron. Dosage should be individualized based on documented deficiency by laboratory tests. Deficiency leads to decreased T-cell counts. Do not take iron supplements unless your doctor has confirmed you are iron deficient.

These dosages are guidelines only, and individual requirements will vary. All vitamin and mineral supplements should be labeled "corn, milk, wheat, soy, sugar, and yeast free." Your doctor or health care professional may have further recommendations depending on your particular needs.

Each of these nutrients is found in a healthy diet of meat, fruits, and vegetables. But under the circumstances of potential intestinal malabsorption, supplemental doses are indicated to improve their availability. Also, in some cases elimination diets result in unintended deficiencies of some nutrients that must be supplemented until the food is reintroduced. It is important that you understand that long-standing food intolerance may result in a number of physiologic disturbances, which must be corrected before you will feel your best. This will take time, but now that you are eating in a healthy manner, you have all the time in the world.

The immune system has been shown to benefit from a variety of activities—music, regular physical exercise, deep breathing exercises, laughter, a positive mental attitude, and regular sleep patterns. Take a minute and look at this list of great ideas that are healthy to boot, and think of ways you can further incorporate them into your life.

Several herbal remedies and tonics may be beneficial to the immune system. For those interested in taking a more active part in their nutritional well-being, the *Encyclopedia of Nutritional Supplements* (1996), by Michael T. Murray, N.D., is an excellent reference. Although laboratory information regarding the exact effects of herbs on the immune system is scarce, enough of us have recognized their healing powers to warrant their inclusion here. Among the common herbs and natural supplements that have a beneficial impact on the immune system are the following:

- Garlic
- Ginseng
- Echinacea
- Astragalus
- Spirulina (actually a food)

Because doses of these products are variable, you may find it helpful to discuss their use with a practitioner who is acquainted with their benefits in order to achieve the best results. The human body contains as many mysteries as there are foods. We'll figure them out later; just get well now. Once you correct nutrient deficiencies and food sensitivities, you are equipped to experience life to the fullest. You may be surprised at how good you feel every day now.

Eating to Avoid Food Intolerance:
Rotate It

Once food sensitivities have occupied a place in your life, you will be eager to avoid them in the future. Although there is no fail-safe method to prevent the development of new food sensitivities, some practical precautions can help. Ideally, planning meals in such a way as to avoid eating the same food more often than every four days is an excellent preventive. This allows your body to recoup its immune forces between exposures, and such rare exposure to the food antigen is unlikely to perpetuate food intolerance. This technique has the added benefit of incorporating a wider variety of foods into the diet for nutrient purposes.

Save Your Enzymes

Using supplemental digestive enzymes may improve your digestion of food. As mentioned earlier, your body will not develop intolerance to the individual amino acids and fatty acids in food. Thorough digestion is without question important in preventing food intolerance. Although digestive enzyme deficiency is common in the elderly, enzyme deficiency may also occur in younger people who overeat.

Our modern diet, composed of highly processed foods, places an enormous demand on our digestive enzymes. These boxed and packaged foods are "dead food." The living, natural enzymes originally present in the food have been killed by processing. This means that the body must bear the entire enzymatic burden for digestion. Eating such food day after day creates a tremendous drain on our digestive resources. Add to this the enormous quantities of food that are commonly consumed with a chew and a swallow in our fast-paced lives, and the digestive enzymes our body has allotted for a meal are soon overwhelmed. This results in large quantities of incompletely digested food entering our intestine for absorption.

This mass of partially digested food is the cornerstone of food intolerance. Any disruption in the integrity of the absorptive surface of the intestine may allow the actual absorption of this undigested food into the bloodstream. However, if the food had been well digested, even less than ideal intestinal conditions would have allowed only well-digested food particles to be absorbed. Because the immune system selectively ignores the small components of well-digested food, allergic reactions mediated by the immune system are avoided.

In the Raw

Eat slowly, chew food well, and eat as much raw food as possible. Raw food retains enzymes that begin assisting in digestion as soon as chewing begins. This improves the efficiency of our own enzymes, because the body only secretes the amount of enzyme needed to completely digest a food. If natural enzymes are present in the food, the body will need to secrete fewer of its own precious enzymes to finish the job.

Raw food, however, contains only enough enzymes for its own digestion. The enzymes of raw food cannot be expected to contribute to the digestion of "dead" or processed food. Use of our enzyme stores for digestion leaves fewer enzymes available to carry out normal metabolic processes, such as tissue repair and detoxification. Once the value of digestive enzymes is appreciated, supplemental enzymes are recognized for the bargain they are. If supplemental enzymes are used, they should be of "pharmaceutical" grade and not the commercial grade found in most health food stores. The AMTL Company, provider of the ALCAT test, has available a high-quality enzyme supplement to benefit those who are food intolerant.

Keep Food Simple

As I have mentioned before, rotating foods is an integral part of avoiding food intolerance. To do this, you must concentrate on eating simple foods—pure, straightforward dishes. Put aside foods blended from many different ingredients for the time being. Eating concoctions that contain a large number of different foods in each dish makes varying foods on a daily basis difficult.

For example, after eating a complicated casserole and salad dinner, you could easily find yourself needing to avoid wheat, corn, tomatoes, milk, chicken, peppers, onions, beans, cheese, rice, eggs, avocados, and brewers yeast for a period of three days. In one fell swoop the next three days' eating is severely limited. Careful planning, however, can yield tasty and well-rounded simple meals for all four days.

Processed Food Is Dead Food

Packaged, highly processed convenience foods resemble their natural namesake only in name. Stripped of nutrients, these foods pose a threat to health because of their tendency to provoke intolerance. The high chemical and preservative content of processed foods qualify them to stay on the shelf—so leave them there. Common sense dictates avoiding these pseudo-foods and returning to foods in their nutritionally rich natural form.

Timing Is Everything

It takes an estimated 20 minutes for the brain to get the message from the stomach that hunger is no longer a problem. This may not sound scientific, but nonetheless it is a simplified version of the feedback mechanisms of hormones released following the absorption of macronutrients (basically fat, carbohydrate, and protein). The body is programmed to assume that when you eat, you are eating naturally occurring foods. In these, the macronutrient is a carrier for various micronutrients, which are the "personality" of your body systems.

Micronutrients include vitamins, minerals, trace elements, coenzymes, and enzymes—all found naturally in unprocessed foods. When provided the appropriate amount of micronutrient, each system operates at its peak efficiency. Deficiencies of micronutrient may result in cravings or hunger. One particularly bizarre example of this is iron deficiency; those who lack sufficient iron may crave substances such as starch, ice, and clay. The physiologic basis of this condition, known as pica, is not understood. However, the fact that a micronutrient deficiency can create an abnormal hunger is thought provoking.

As mentioned earlier, the recognized feedback mechanisms for hunger depend on intake of macronutrient. Allowing the body the necessary time to digest and absorb macronutrient to satisfy hunger is crucial. It takes about 20 minutes for the "no-longer-hungry" or satiety signal to get from the stomach to the brain. And we all know how much damage can be done to a plate of food in 20 minutes. Macronutrient, as previously defined, is the body's source of calories. It is also the body's source of allergic reactions. I know of no research suggesting allergic reactions resulting from naturally occurring vitamins or minerals (micronutrient). At any rate, allowing at least 20 minutes for eating allows your enzymatic digestion to keep pace and stopping eating when your hunger subsides prevents overtaxing the digestive capacity. Get in the habit of leaving food on the plate.

Water, Water Everywhere, and Not Enough Is Drunk

Water is the elixir of youth. It serves more functions in the body than a secretary in a busy real-estate office. Drinking water helps fill the stomach and decrease hunger. While washing waste out of the intestine as a natural laxative, water also maintains the integrity of the cardiovascular system, speeds the removal of waste and toxins through the liver and kidneys, enhances the appearance of skin, and functions in innumerable chemical reactions in the body. Water dilutes adverse chemical reactions in the bloodstream and speeds their elimination; it also hydrates the skin and mucous membranes, including the intestinal lining. A person may live an estimated 30 days without food, but only three days without water. Recognize its importance to you, and drink water instead of chemical liquid convenience drinks.

Recognize its importance to you, and drink water instead of chemical liquid convenience drinks.

There is much controversy regarding the safety of different water supplies. Chlorine is an excellent additive to water until it reaches your lips. As you increase your water intake, use filtered water or bottled spring water to minimize exposure to unnecessary chemicals. These sources are not unconditionally safe, but overall are a better choice, in my opinion, than chlorinated water.

The chlorine in municipal water supplies is toxic to the beneficial bacteria of the intestines. These bacteria perform important digestive functions for us in exchange for a place to live. Undue elimination of these bacteria may increase the likelihood that yeast will colonize in the intestines. These parasites may disturb absorption and predispose us to food intolerance by virtue of their effect on the intestinal lining.

Drink between two and three liters of water a day to supply the body with all it needs for a full day's work. If you have unusual conditions such as congestive heart failure or kidney disease, ask your doctor before increasing your water intake. But even with such conditions, sodas, coffee, and tea are not substitutes for pure water.

When Intolerant, Do as Intolerants Do

If you are intolerant of a food, take a proactive stance in avoiding it. It doesn't matter whether you eat a reactive food intentionally or out of ignorance; the results will be the same. Knowledge is power, but knowledge is impotent unless implemented. Once you know your reactive foods, use this greater power to control your health.

Don't Mess with Mother Intestine

The rate-limiting factor in the development of food intolerance is the intestinal lining. As long as it is intact and functioning properly, food intolerance is less likely to develop. Because food intolerance usually involves the body's immune system recognizing a food particle as foreign, absorbing only completely digested food across the intestinal lining precludes most adverse reactions to foods, except those that are pharmacologically mediated or toxic. As mentioned previously, the immune system will not react to individual amino acids, fatty acids, or very small carbohydrate particles.

Avoid unnecessary doses of aspirin and nonsteroid anti-inflammatory drugs (NSAIDs), because they have a direct effect on the intestinal wall and may predispose you to food intolerance. Overindulging in alcoholic beverages is known to irritate the gastrointestinal tract. Overusing antibiotics will disrupt the natural balance of gut flora. Anything that disturbs your intestine, in fact, may predispose you to food intolerance.

Synopsis

1. Medical professionals have known for years that patients who eliminate allergenic foods from their diet lose weight.

2. Individual doctors confirm the benefits of ALCAT testing for their patients.

3. Food intolerance results in inflammatory reactions mediated by the immune system.

4. Everyone is an individual as far as their biochemistry is concerned. No one diet will work well for everyone; they must identify and eliminate foods to which they react.

5. The ALCAT test is a simple blood test that determines foods to which you react as well as those that are safe to eat.

6. Certain supplements may enhance immune system function as you embark on an elimination diet.

7. Following the ALCAT food plan eat simple raw foods, eat slowly, take digestive enzymes, and drink plenty of safe water.

CHAPTER 10

Airways and
Food Intolerance

There is no feeling more terrifying than running out of oxygen. Allergic airway disease may be due to food intolerance as well as airborne allergens. Yet of conditions traditional doctors believe are *not* helped by addressing a person's food intolerance, airway problems—including asthma, hay fever, and sinusitis—top the list. The general belief is that these conditions are caused almost exclusively by inhalant allergies. But as already mentioned, nothing is simple in the world of allergy and food intolerance. By excluding a diagnosis of food intolerance from the possible causes of respiratory ailments, physicians could be allowing several million people to suffer more than is necessary each year.

Breathing Easier

But luckily for many people, some doctors do take the link between food and respiratory problems into consideration.

Gretchen, Moselle, Patricia, Christian, and Stacey, whose cases are given below, are a few people who now breathe easier because their doctors recognize the powerful impact food intolerance can have on any illness, including respiratory problems. Groundbreaking research is also showing that testing for food intolerance is a promising therapy for the millions who suffer from respiratory problems, and who long to breathe easier once again.

Enjoying Springtime for the First Time

Gretchen is among the grateful former sinus sufferers who lived for years with hay fever and asthma. She was so happy to be free of a dripping nose, stuffy sinus, and labored breathing spells that she wrote to thank Just Hintz, the director of an ALCAT Testing Laboratory in Germany, for helping her regain her health.

> I would like to thank you for what you have given me with your allergy test. You've given me symptom-free springs. In previous years, I suffered in the most beautiful time of the year with very aggressive hay fever which kept me awake for many nights and which was also the origin of my asthma. Since I was not able to breathe well on my own, an inhalator was my constant partner. Therapeutic nose drops didn't bring any relief. The worst part of my condition was not being able to breathe and the helplessness of not being able to do anything about it.
>
> I could not accept this helplessness and I started reading about allergies. Quickly, I realized that it was not only the pollen that could be causing my suffering, but food allergy could also be the origin of my symptoms. In my research, I read about your ALCAT Test, and after giving it careful thought, I decided to do the test. I can only say, thank God. Since avoiding the foods to which I'm allergic, including the most severe—grains—I have no more symptoms. I'm reminded of the benefit of the test every time I cheat on my diet. For example, if I take even a little bite of a roll at Sunday breakfast, for the next two days I'll have a dripping nose.

Like many people, Gretchen was one of the lucky hay fever and asthma suffers who learned that foods were either causing or exacerbating her respiratory problems. Unfortunately, millions of others have not yet been tested for the possibility. "Because this relationship between food and the nose is not widely recognized by most conventional doctors, few patients with this problem get satisfactory treatment," wrote Dr. Jonathan Brostoff in his book *Hay Fever: The Complete Guide.* "And because the symptoms do not come on as soon as they eat the food, the patients themselves are generally unaware of the connection." He agrees that food intolerance is worth considering as a therapy for people suffering from respiratory problems, considering the growing numbers of people who are already being helped.

The Breath of Life

Moselle doesn't even want to think about where she would be today if a doctor hadn't finally diagnosed food intolerance as the cause of her recurrent sinusitis, a condition she'd suffered for five years. The chronic sinus condition had become particularly severe following a bad cold and a ruptured eardrum in 1984. Within months, her health deteriorated to the point that she had to quit her job as a registered nurse. So fatigued by her condition that she didn't have the energy to take care of her house any longer, she was also forced to move from her beloved home into a small condominium. "I couldn't keep up with the everyday activities of living," she explains. Over five years, Moselle saw three ear, nose, and throat specialists, and she was constantly on antibiotics. "As soon as the effect of one antibiotic wore off, I would get another sinus infection." At one point she was even in the hospital for ten days on intravenous penicillin. She also had to have surgery to fix a deviated septum that developed from her affliction.

Despite all these medical treatments, Moselle's health continued a downhill slide—until the day she visited Dr. Barbara Solomon and was tested for food intolerance. Moselle explains:

It turned my whole life around. I had tried to address my sinus condition through conventional means and mainstream doctors. They experimented with all sorts of methods on me, but since none of the treatments were working I'd gotten to the point that I believed I was going to have to live for the rest of my life with breathing problems, headaches, and fatigue. I was very skeptical when I first came to Dr. Solomon and she told me that she thought she could help me, because all of the other doctors had said they could help me, too. The first thing she addressed was food allergy, which was very foreign to me. But I went on a diet that eliminated all of my food allergens, including corn, wheat, yeast, sugar, and milk, and I was better almost immediately. Within a year I started looking for a new home. With my health back, the condominium had become too boring. Now I'm able to do gardening again and do all of the things I love doing. I even took a part-time nursing job—with Dr. Solomon.

The Trouble with Asthma

Asthma, hay fever, and sinusitis are among the most common allergy complaints today. Asthma, in particular, is on the rise. This potentially dangerous disease is thought to be compounded by our increasingly polluted and chemically adulterated modern world. Twelve million people suffer from asthma in the United States alone. Of these, five thousand die every year. In fact, mortality has doubled since 1978, with people who live in cities being the hardest hit. The characteristic symptoms of asthma, which include wheezing, coughing, shortness of breath, and chest tightness, are produced by a constriction of the air passages.

This happens when an allergen triggers IgE antibodies in the mast cells of the bronchial tubes, which lead from the trachea to the lungs. The antibodies cause the mast cells to release their powerful chemicals—including the well-known chemical mediator histamine. This causes inflammation of the membranes lining the tubes. The tubes then become thicker and produce more mucus, which restricts the passage of air. A full-blown asthma attack occurs when so many chemicals are released from the mast cells that the smooth muscles of the bronchial tubes contract and become narrow, making a fresh breath of air increasingly difficult.

Today's medical treatments for asthma are surprisingly disappointing, considering asthma's prevalence and rate of growth. Therapy typically involves a series of drugs including bronchodilators and anti-inflammatories. However, among the drawbacks of these medications are their short-lived effects and serious side effects, including fogginess, fatigue, even death. Long-term use of steroids poses serious risk of adrenal suppression and other complications, including weight gain. As in many conditions the response of modern medicine to asthma leaves the sufferer contemplating this question: Is the cure worse than the disease?

Common Airway Conditions

Along with asthma, two other respiratory conditions—hay fever (also known as allergic rhinitis) and sinusitis—are common. Combined, these two respiratory conditions affect an estimated 14 million Americans. Hay fever, which is caused by pollens such as ragweed, affects as many as one in five Americans. In hay fever sufferers, pollen triggers the mast cells of the tissues that come into contact with the environment (including the nose, throat, and eyes) by releasing mediators that cause inflammation of the delicate tissues. Sufferers experience this reaction as red, itchy, watery eyes, and a runny or congested nose. Although usually seasonal, affecting a person when his particular allergen or allergens are in season, hay fever can also be exacerbated by food.

Sinusitis is an unpleasant and often painful infection of the air-filled bony cavities that surround the nasal passages. It is caused by the inflammation that occurs with hay fever and the common cold. The main symptoms of sinusitis are a severely blocked nose, headache over the eyes, or an ache in the cheeks. For some people, like Moselle, a severe case of sinusitis can completely decimate their quality of life.

Food intolerance triggers the body by different mechanisms than traditional airborne and traditional food allergy. One theory is that in a person with food intolerance the food allergen, combined with an airborne allergy, puts additional stress on the body and it collapses under the load, such as Moselle did.

Identifying the Thieves of Good Health

Of course, like Moselle, some lucky people find that by avoiding their intolerant foods, they find a cure for their airway conditions, or at the very least, reduce the impact of their problems. Like Moselle, Patricia was stunned to learn that the very foods she ate every day were ruining her health. She had suffered for years with asthma and eczema, when she finally found Dr. John W. Gerrard, an allergy and immunology specialist and former Professor of Pediatrics at the University of Saskatchewan in Canada. Although she suffered extensively from both conditions, she never associated the onset of a bout of asthma or skin rash with the particular foods she was eating. In fact, she says that if she'd had to guess which foods were aggravating her health problems, she would never have presumed that apples, oranges, broccoli, and tomatoes would be on the list.

But it wasn't until she eliminated those foods, as well as many others, that she was cured of the eczema for the first time in her life and helped tremendously with her asthma. "Once I began eliminating the foods, my system cleared up, and I was able to identify exactly which foods were triggering the asthma," she explains. "Now, I can't even go near a jar of peanut butter without my lungs getting congested."

Food intolerance is a promising therapy for the millions . . . who long to breathe easier once again.

Christian Mayer (see "World Class Health" in chapter 1) is also among the benefactors of the attention given to the relationship between food intolerance and respiratory problems. This world-class Austrian skier, who won the World Cup in the Giant Slalom two years in a row and a bronze medal at the Winter Olympics in Lillehammer, suffered every season with breathing problems. The stuffy air in airplanes and hotels exacerbated his condition when he had to travel to competitions. Needless to say, his coach was not happy about having one of his top skiers waylaid by a health problem. He sent Christian to an Austrian physician, Dr. Stephen Shimpf, who specializes in immunotherapy and preventative medicine in Salzburg.

As he does with many of his patients, Dr. Shimpf tested Christian for food intolerance using the ALCAT Test. The results of the blood test showed that the skier was intolerant to rice, milk products, wheat, apples, bananas, and beer, most of which he consumed every day. Once he removed those foods his stuffy nose cleared up. In addition, he was able to avoid (unlike some of his team members) the usual seasonal colds and flu. As an added bonus he lost the extra ten pounds he typically gained in the off-season and he had more energy. But this world-class athlete says the most important benefit is this: "I'm winning. Right after the test I won my first World Cup in America. I was surprised by the test results because I'd always thought foods like apples and bananas are healthy, but they're not for me. I avoid my reactive foods and I feel better."

Dr. Shimpf, however, was not surprised by the results. "I've gotten used to great results with food intolerance testing with my patients, so amazing results like this no longer astonish me." He has found food intolerance testing to be a big help in treating patients who suffer from respiratory conditions among other problems. Besides Christian, Dr. Shimpf points to a particularly "interesting case" of a 30-year-old woman who had endured severe asthma for years. After he tested her blood and she eliminated her reactive foods for three to four months, she was able to significantly reduce her intake of cortisone, which she'd been taking for years to deal with debilitating asthma attacks. "This reduction of intake of a pharmaceutical as strong as cortisone alone had an additional positive impact on her health," notes Schimpf.

A Promising Treatment for Millions

Many other respiratory sufferers around the world have duplicated the improvement of Moselle, Christian, and Patricia—thanks to eliminating intolerant foods from their diets. Several research studies have also shown that food does indeed have a significant impact on airway conditions. These findings clearly show a promising treatment for the millions around the world who long to breathe free once again.

Among the many interesting research results on the effects of food intolerance and respiratory health problems are the findings of two studies conducted by Drs. Peter Fell and Jonathan Brostoff. Both studies are based on the results of testing people for food intolerance using the ALCAT Test. In the first study, conducted in 1988, Drs. Fell and Brostoff reported that all eight patients who had suffered for more than three years with hay fever were successful in reducing or eliminating their upper respiratory symptoms. The researchers reported that although many of these patients were skeptical that their condition had a dietary cause, the results were clear-cut improvements due to the elimination of reactive foods. By sticking to their ALCAT-designed diets, patients maintained positive results through their follow-up exams.

In a second study conducted in 1990, Drs. Fell and Brostoff found slightly less dramatic results for patients with asthma and rhinitis, but nonetheless significant to the many people seeking non-pharmaceutical treatments to their chronic upper airways diseases. Of the patients studied, whose symptoms included sneezing, running noses, coughing, wheezing, and headaches, four of the 17 completely improved and maintained their improvement with a change in diet and only an occasional need for an accompanying treatment such as a medication or inhalers. The study's authors note that these results are not surprising considering that inhalant allergens also play a major role in these conditions.

Dr. Solomon also found mixed, but overall hopeful, results in her study of 172 patients with 11 different conditions. Among them were 20 patients with recurrent sinusitis, 108 patients with hay fever, and 18 patients with asthma. All the patients were put on diets that eliminated their allergenic foods. Within a ten-month period, Dr. Solomon found that with diet alone, 59 percent of the people with recurrent sinusitis improved, 42 percent of the patients with hay fever improved, and 30 percent of the patients with asthma improved.

Many other studies have found that food allergy is an important cause of asthma and hay fever. Among them are two relatively recent studies, including one in 1987 by Zdenek Pelikan, director of the Department of Allergy and Immunology at the Institute of Medical Sciences in the Netherlands. Pelikan investigated the role of food allergy in patients with rhinitis, some of whom had accompanying symptoms of sinusitis and headache. He found that the role of foods was confirmed in two-thirds of the patients with hay fever where an allergic component was suspected. Further, in 19 percent of these cases, food was found to be the sole cause of the patients' hay fever. In half these patients, the hay fever was caused by various inhalant allergens with foods also having an effect (known as "secondary" food allergy). Pelikan commented that "the role of food allergy and of food in general in subjects with allergic disorders, especially in those suffering from rhinitis, otitis media, and sinusitis, is still underestimated by clinicians."

In the second study, Dr. D. G. Wraith, consultant physician with the Allergy Clinic in London, tested several aspects of food intolerance in a number of patients with asthma in 1987 and concluded that "food allergy is very important cause of asthma but is often overlooked." Further, he reported, "Avoidance of the cause would prevent much disability and also lessen the amount of drugs needed, which is important considering their expense and potential side-effects."

These studies are just a few of the many going back several decades that clearly point to the relationship of food intolerance to respiratory conditions, including food intolerance in children as young as newborns. For example, Dr. John Gerrard found a clear relationship between cow's milk and infants in two of his studies, entitled "Food-Induced Respiratory Disease" and "Familial Recurrent Rhinorrhea and Bronchitis Due to Cow's Milk," conducted in 1966.

Hope for a Healthy Future

The dramatically high number of respiratory sufferers is not surprising considering the complex and sensitive respiratory system. It includes miles of air passages in the lungs. By the time air reaches these passages, it has already been warmed and moistened by the nose, filtered through nose hairs and lymph tissue in the throat, and then re-filtered by millions of tiny cilia (hair-like projections along membranous cell tissue) to remove any particles that could damage the lungs.

Unfortunately for Stacey, this complex respiratory system broke down so severely that she had to have one lung removed. A downward spiral in her health quickly followed lung cancer surgery. Stacey developed pneumonia in her other lung and couldn't speak above a whisper and without extreme effort for nearly a year. She began seeing any medical practitioner who would give her any bit of hope. A chiropractor she was seeing recommended a dietitian who worked extensively in the area of food intolerance. The dietitian immediately had Stacey tested for food allergies using the ALCAT blood test. "The test was terrific," says Stacey. "It showed me the foods I was allergic to, and the minute I started eating only what the test indicated was safe for me to eat, I was able to speak without gasping for air. I speak beautifully now."

Like Patricia, Stacey showed intolerance to a long list of foods that she never would have suspected without a specific test. She can no longer eat many vegetables she used to enjoy, including everything *but* spinach, broccoli, green beans, and cabbage. She's also not able to eat condiments such as garlic, oregano, vanilla, and cinnamon. "Those are things I never would have guessed in a million years that my body couldn't tolerate. And without the test, I never would have believed that the vegetables I loved so much were killing me. Ironically, other doctors had told me to eat healthier, including eating all the vegetables I wanted. They didn't have a clue that those vegetables were helping to make me sick. I am so grateful for this test."

Stacey is among a growing number of people who were victims of inhalant allergies for years before finding a doctor who was experienced in finding the source of respiratory problems by testing a patient's blood against a battery of food allergens. The ALCAT Test also tests for sensitivities to molds and chemicals such as preservatives and food dyes—all of which can contribute either directly or indirectly to respiratory difficulties. As many practitioners believe, these intolerances represent more load on the body, and the air passages are a likely target for a system weakened by the elements.

CHAPTER 11

Skin and Food Intolerance

Imagine being completely uncomfortable in your own skin. That is a fact of life for millions who suffer from skin conditions such as eczema, urticaria, angioedema, and severe acne. Yet much of the suffering due to these puzzling skin conditions could be prevented through elimination of reactive foods. Even cellulite, the scourge of women everywhere, is closely associated with food intolerance.

Eczema and Food Sensitivities

It's a fact of life for people like Patricia, who at 26 had suffered for years with raw patches of itchy, blistered eczema from head to toe. (Patricia also suffered from asthma—see previous chapter.) Eczema, one of the most common skin conditions, is an inflammation of the outer layer of skin which, in the early stages, may be red, blistered, swollen, weeping, and extremely itchy. Later, usually after much scratching by the sufferer, it becomes crusted, scaly, and thickened. Patricia's skin was so sensitive that she had many sleepless nights. Everything irritated her raw skin, including the blankets, sheets, pillows, and pajamas. During the day her clothes irritated her skin.

Finally, the unbearable pain forced her to quit her job. After years of suffering and trying all kinds of therapies recommended by a variety of doctors, hopeless and in pain, she ended up at allergy and immunology specialist Dr. John Gerrard's office in Saskatchewan, Canada. He saw that she was a good candidate for food intolerance, because her eczema had gone away during a period when she had pneumonia and couldn't eat. The ALCAT Test identified so many reactive foods that she was left to eat only a few vegetables, a few fruits, and some organically raised meat. As soon as she eliminated her reactive foods, her eczema cleared up right away. "Without this test I would have never known foods were aggravating my eczema. This test identified which foods bothered me."

Virginia, another person suffering from eczema, says that since childhood she'd had problems with allergies and eczema, and that when she was 18, the eczema suddenly got worse, then went downhill from there. With her first pregnancy, her skin "went totally wild." Her diet is so limited now that she has to be very careful with her meals. She eats seasonal foods as much as possible and rotates the foods to which she has no sensitivity. Whenever she grows lax with her meals, she immediately starts itching again. "Even one bite of apple makes me itchy. And if I eat beef my skin gets raw."

Virginia's story is not the only extreme case of a skin condition that responded well to food intolerance testing. Thousands of patients—both adults and children—are enjoying healthy skin, free of irritations, by eliminating foods to which they showed intolerance. However, while traditional medicine recognizes food allergy if the result is an *immediate* skin rash, when the reaction is delayed, as it often is in food intolerance, traditional doctors tend to ignore the possibility of food sensitivity as a cause of the skin problems. This is true despite success stories like Virginia's and many research studies by respected medical professionals. "Early in my career I learned that careful dietary histories are important in treating patients and that ordinary, healthy foods can cause many problems, including skin conditions," says Dr. Gerrard, former professor of Pediatrics at the University of Saskatchewan, Canada. He has conducted a great deal of research on the topic. "It's a great disappointment that doctors just don't bother to consider food intolerance, because foods can be so helpful with so many different problems."

Itching to Be Allergic

"Many controversies exist about the nature and importance of adverse reactions to food and chemical additives to human diseases, and the whole spectrum of symptoms that may appear are not delineated," explains Lene Høj, a Danish doctor of internal medicine and specialist in allergic diseases. "But my success in treating patients and my research in the area of food intolerance clearly shows that a long list of conditions and symptoms are related to food allergies including eczema and urticaria." One of the most severe skin conditions that Dr. Høj has seen in her 17 years in practice as an allergy specialist in Denmark was a four-year-old boy named Henry, whose skin was so covered in rashes, scars, and wounds that he was tormented day and night by itching. It seemed that no matter what Henry's mother tried, her son's condition only got worse.

His suffering began when his mother stopped breast-feeding him and put him on commercial formula. An itching rash began appearing on his face and arms, and his constant scratching left the skin raw and bloody. When his mother put gloves on his hands to try and prevent him from scratching his wounds, he would rub his skin against carpets and on furniture. He looked so different from other children his age that he became withdrawn, developed learning disabilities, and began having suicidal thoughts. After seeing a battery of doctors, Henry was using six types of allergy medications and a special skin cream, which did little to ease his physical pain.

Dr. Høj tested him for food and chemical sensitivities using the ALCAT Test and found Henry had many allergies. His mother began carefully preparing his daily meals, which consisted of lowfat yogurt without sugar for breakfast, and whole-grain rye bread and ham, tuna fish, or specially made liver paté without bacon for lunch. Finally, his condition was under control, his skin cleared up, and Henry began picking up where his life left off. The condition took its toll psychologically, but today he goes to school with other children who have developmental problems. He now has a job, but has to wear special gloves so that his skin is protected from irritants like dust. Henry's mother doesn't mind the daily preparation of food, which includes making all the meals from scratch. She's just glad that her son is able to live a somewhat normal life.

With regards to food allergy and skin conditions, Høj explains that when allergy is the root of eczema and urticaria, the mast cells in the lower layers of the skin are believed to cause the problem. When they degranulate, the mediators that are released have a powerful effect on the capillaries (tiny blood vessels) that lie all around them in the skin. These capillaries become leakier, allowing plasma (the watery part of the blood) to seep out into the skin itself. This produces the characteristic swellings and itchiness of urticaria, which is a skin disruption with temporary welts of various shapes and sizes with clear margins and pale centers. Urticaria is often thought to be triggered by food, drugs, and stress. Sometimes it's triggered by cold. Where a great deal of seepage from the blood vessels occurs, the tissues below the skin may also become filled with watery fluid. This produces a puffiness that doctors describe as localized angioedema (or edema), an abnormal pooling of fluid in the tissues.

A Child's Pain Is Everyone's Pain

When a child is in pain, parents suffer as much or more than the child does. So you can imagine their relief to find a correct diagnosis of food intolerance after years of futile medical treatments. A mother in Germany wrote to Mr. Just Hintz, laboratory manager in Hamburg, Germany, after finally finding the solution to her daughter's suffering:

> I am sending a few lines to express my thanks and appreciation to you. No doctor was able to help my daughter, who suffered severely from neurodermatitis. In June 1990, we came to your office the first time. Sarah, who was born in February 1985, was six months old when she developed red, itchy skin. After seeing several doctors, she was diagnosed with neurodermatitis, and treated for five years with cortisone cream. These creams did not bring about any healing, only some short-term relief.
>
> In the meantime, the disease had increased to the point that our whole family was suffering, both physically and psychologically. No one could get a good night's sleep; we felt sick right along with Sarah. She lived with a constant, strong urge to scratch, and whenever she scratched her whole body would be full of scabs and open wounds. She had all of the classic symptoms, which are very well known to the medical community. But what is not well

known is the method you used to treat her condition. When she was tested for food intolerance in June 1990, we were told with great astonishment the foods that Sarah is reacting to allergically.

At the beginning, we were shocked, wondering how we could handle all of this. Her whole diet had to be changed, including no more rye and sugar; several spices and vegetables had to go away if we wanted to have success. Now, three years later we are so happy that all these efforts have paid off. Her new diet was a complete success for every one of us, but mainly for Sarah, who had suffered for so long. Seeing her perfectly smooth skin now, it seems like a miracle.

Hives and Food Intolerance

In traditional medicine, skin rashes such as eczema and urticaria are believed to be predominantly a problem among children. But as Virginia's and others' stories point out, adults are not excepted from these conditions. Shortly after starting a new job as a banker in the fall of 1995, Frank came down with bronchitis. Knowing he was allergic to penicillin, his doctors put him on another antibiotic. He woke up just days later with hives all over his body and big painful blisters on his face and head. His doctor diagnosed urticaria.

No matter what Frank tried or what his doctors prescribed, the hives didn't go away or even improve. Finally, at the suggestion of a co-worker, he made an appointment with Dr. Barbara Solomon. After listening to his medical history, she recommended an ALCAT Test. He showed intolerance to several foods including sugar, wheat, corn, pork, and some fish. After eliminating those foods, as best as he could in his busy career as a banker, his condition improved to a manageable level.

Ironically, shortly after that, his wife was hospitalized for a heart condition. Her second day in the hospital, Patsy broke out in a rash and was swollen from head to toe. "I was one big, swollen sore all over my body." Her family doctor diagnosed angioedema. Many conditions can cause angioedema, such as heart or kidney failure and allergic reactions. He thought that it was an allergy to something, but never guessed that the food she was given in the hospital was the cause. Dr. Solomon tested her and found allergies to several foods, including chicken, potatoes, and green beans—the very foods she'd been fed in the hospital the night before her skin broke out. By eliminating their intolerant foods, she and her husband were able to get relief from the hives and blisters, as well as improve their overall health and lose several pounds of excess weight.

Acne Relief with Food Elimination

Allergy testing is not just for severe skin conditions. Many people have had success at clearing up acne, especially as a side effect of eliminating intolerant foods for other medical conditions. Brenda, a banker in her early 40s, for example, had an ALCAT Test done to improve her overall health. She had few food intolerances, but one of her primary sensitivities was to cinnamon. After eliminating the spice, her chronic acne cleared up completely.

As shown with these patient case histories, there is no effective way to diagnose food intolerance for each person without individual testing. Guesswork alone will not help most people find out which foods, chemicals, and other substances they should not eat. While one person can eat chicken, like Patsy's husband, others such as

Patsy herself cannot. One person, like Henry, can eat rye but not wheat; another, like Sarah, breaks out if she eats rye. Despite success stories like these, you'll find few traditional allergy doctors who would agree that delayed food reactions cause skin conditions.

One of the problems in their lack of acceptance of this therapy is that many current research studies on food intolerance and skin conditions show just over 50 percent improvement—which many do not believe is statistically significant. These studies may not show results as high as those of other studies on food intolerance and conditions such as migraine, fatigue, and weight loss. But 50 percent improvement does show nonetheless that food intolerance is clearly a viable therapy for at least half of the millions of people who suffer from painful skin irritations. It means that the Virginias, Franks, Sarahs, and Patsys in the world get their chance to live a pain-free life.

In several research studies on the ALCAT Test, doctors found over 50 percent improvement in eczema, urticaria, angioedema, and general skin condition by eliminating specific food intolerances. In their 1988 study on the ALCAT Test, Drs. Fell and Brostoff found that patients with eczema and urticaria who stuck to their ALCAT diets improved over a six-week period. In a second study in 1990 on the effectiveness of the ALCAT Test in treating four common patient complaints, Drs. Fell and Brostoff found that after one year 26 patients (9 with urticaria and 17 with eczema) improved by an estimated 50 percent. The nine urticaria patients showed a striking improvement—two completely resolved and six maintained their success rate over the course of the 12-month study.

Consistent with this percentage, Dr. Barbara Solomon reported in 1992 that 11 patients with eczema improved by 55 percent when they eliminated their intolerant foods.

Further, J. R. Cabo-Soler, M.D., a medical faculty member and chief of the Biochemistry Department at the University of Valencia in Spain, noted that in addition to losing weight, patients also reported greater quality to their skin— more smoothness and less dryness and flaking,

Eczema Improves with Weight Loss

In a one-month study on the relationship of food intolerance to weight loss, body composition, and self-reported disease symptoms conducted in 1995 at the Columbia/ HCA Medical Center's Sports Medicine and Performance Center in Houston, lead investigator Gilbert Kaats, Ph.D., found a much higher than 50 percent improvement in eczema symptoms after patients followed a diet that eliminated their intolerant foods. In fact, the individuals in the experimental group (50 participants) who had reported problems with eczema averaged a 66 percent improvement in their skin condition after following the diet.

On the other hand, those in the control group (50 individuals) who reported eczema problems said that their skin condition got about 33 percent *worse* after following diets of their own choosing. Interestingly, both groups reported nearly the same level of skin trouble at the beginning of study. "While the individuals on the ALCAT diet consistently performed better than the control group in all disease-symptom categories, eczema was the only condition in which the control group actually reported *worse* symptoms while on diets of their own choosing," said Dr. Kaats, director of the Health and Medical Research Foundation, an independent research organization in San Antonio.

Reactive Foods Get Under Your Skin

For the past several decades many researchers from around the world, all known for their special interest in atopic eczema, have independently described the value of food intolerance as a therapy for chronic skin conditions. Among them, Dr. Albert Rowe in 1951 found a correlation between food allergies and atopic dermatitis in infants and children. In 1966, Dr. G. Hagerman examined the importance of food factors in atopic dermatitis. In 1978, Dr. P. Juto found a strict elimination diet effective in the treatment of infantile atopic eczema. Michael Pike, Research Fellow, Institute of Child Health, London, found a measurable improvement in skin problems using elimination diets. He said:

> These data do provide evidence that, in at least some individuals with atopic eczema, ingestion of certain foods will provoke a reaction of some kind, be it eczematous or urticaria. We are often asked by skeptical [sic] colleagues, "Do you really believe all this 'food business'?" It remains one of the sadder aspects of mainstream medicine that we should see such an important problem as a question of "belief" or "non-belief." What is actually needed is an open, inquiring attitude, and careful, critical investigation. By failing to study the relationship between foods and atopic eczema, we might deny ourselves the opportunity of understanding and thus eventually overcoming this common and distressing disease.

Medical experts who recognize food intolerance believe in this therapy as an effective option for many skin condition sufferers. "There is growing evidence that what goes into the mouth can produce a reaction in the skin, and that food is an important factor," says Dr. Brostoff.

Dr. Stephen Schimpf, the preventive medicine and immunotherapy doctor who treated Austria's Olympic skiers, said that by eliminating intolerant foods, in accordance with test results, one patient with severe psoriasis was cured of all his allergic-like symptoms including severe itching and skin so hot at night that he couldn't sleep. "Now he's able to get a good night's sleep. We've seen many patients' allergic-like symptoms go away when they eliminate their allergenic foods."

Dr. I. A. Schapkaitz, a general practitioner in Johannesburg, South Africa, found the ALCAT Test a great help in his practice, in particular with eczema and urticaria. "When you've had a patient with severe urticaria who has suffered for months on end, and you put them on an ALCAT diet and see them get better, as a physician it's very gratifying and rewarding."

Cellulite—Such a Pretty Name

No discussion of fat or overweight would be complete without some reference to cellulite. This anatomical eyesore, which very much affects the appearance of skin, has become the dread of every woman in a bathing suit. So poorly understood, and yet so hated, cellulite is the result of modern lifestyles to a great extent. According to Dr. Elizabeth Dancey in her book *The Cellulite Solution,* "95% of women have or believe they have cellulite."

It is hard to believe that there is as yet no known cure for a condition that affects such a large segment of the population. Because no established medical treatment protocol exists, most physicians avoid treating cellulite. This opens the way for any number of unscrupulous purveyors of potions to make their pitch to a captive audience of sufferers. To opportunistic entrepreneurs, *cellulite* means "sell you a lot." Interestingly, these potions are not held to the same demanding standards as drugs because they are not applied as a medical intervention. Sales are soaring.

Cellulite is found only in fatty tissue (no one has ever had cellulite in muscle or bone!). But one does not have to be overweight to have cellulite. Cellulite in women most frequently appears on the hips, buttocks, and thighs. Men will tend to develop cellulite on the upper body.

Even cellulite, the scourge of women everywhere, is associated with food intolerance.

Fat storage in the body is controlled by special receptors in each fat cell. These receptors are called alpha2 receptors. Various hormones may stimulate alpha2 receptors and open the doors into the fat cell to allow the deposit of more fat into the cell. The most prominent of these hormones is insulin. Insulin in the blood encourages more fat to be deposited into storage.

On the other hand, beta-receptors open the figurative back door of the fat cells to allow fat out into the bloodstream. Hormones that stimulate the beta-receptors are thyroxin and adrenaline.

As Dr. Dancey poignantly points out in her book, "not all fat is created equal." In women the fat cells around the hips, thighs, and buttocks have six times as many alpha2 receptors as beta-receptors. This implies that fat can be stored six times as fast as it can be released from these areas. Many women will attest to this truth. Elsewhere in the body there are six times as many beta-receptors as alpha2 receptors. This means fat will be lost six times as fast from these areas. Therefore, physiologically, if fat is to be gained, it will most likely show in the hips, thighs, and buttocks. And when fat is lost, it will come from the upper body in most women. This is truly the worst of both worlds and explains a lot. No matter the reason for the weight gain, the overweight will appear on the hips, thighs, and buttocks of most women and on the upper body on men.

Most important to the issues discussed in this book is the high incidence of cellulite in individuals with food intolerance. It seems that food intolerance and its resultant fluid retention, caused by immune-mediated damage to blood vessels, may be a significant contributor to the appearance of cellulite. Those who successfully identify and treat food intolerance may notice an improvement in cellulite. Likewise, quite often those with cellulite may suspect food intolerance. Cellulite may be prevented by the prompt elimination of food intolerance, improvement of lymphatic drainage, and the regeneration of blood supply to these areas of compromised blood supply.

Cellulite actually describes fatty tissue in various stages of development. The word *cellulite* refers to the dimpling appearance of the skin associated with the more advanced stages of change in the subcutaneous fat. Although areas of advanced and long-standing fatty deterioration may be irreparable, much cellulite is actually tissue in a dynamic state of evolution. The latter is amenable to revitalization.

Treatment of cellulite begins with the reversal of adverse physiological changes that predispose to the deterioration of subcutaneous fat. Once the evolution of cellulite is halted, attention may turn to the reversal of body physiology that sustains existing cellulitic tissue. Remember that fatty tissue by its nature and purpose is in a continual state of active change. Successful control of the appearance of cellulite will require ongoing attention to avoiding the negative lifestyle factors that predispose cellulite. A thorough cellulite treatment program will include identification and elimination of food intolerance. Until intolerant foods are eliminated, any improvement in cellulite appearance will be temporary, as cellulite will continue to develop due to deterioration of the circulation in these fatty areas. Once the food sensitivities are eliminated, special efforts to improve circulation and lymphatic drainage in these areas may proceed. The most effective maintenance of healthy tissue appearance is achieved through healthy eating habits:

- **Avoid processed and packaged foods.** These foods are stripped of nutrient value and filled with chemicals to prolong shelf life. They are often rich in simple carbohydrates and fats and tend to cause insulin levels to soar. This results in the prompt storing of the empty fat calories as fat on your body. (Remember, they are six times more likely to be stored as fat in the hips, thighs, and buttocks in women.)

- **Drink at least two and preferably three quarts of fresh water each day.** This should be filtered or bottled spring water to avoid the unpleasant effects of large doses of chlorine on the intestinal bacteria. Also, a fairly large number of people, especially asthmatics, are sensitive to chlorine.

- **Limit caffeine.** Two cups of coffee per day should be the limit. You may also be sensitive to caffeine, however.

- **Avoid alcoholic beverages.** Notwithstanding their possible beneficial effect on heart function when consumed in moderation, these empty calories are destined for your fat bank, which ironically is a strain on your heart.

- **Avoid foods with high salt content.** These foods promote fluid retention and contribute to cellulite.

Some other helpful suggestions in addition to eating tips include:

- **Establish a daily lower body aerobic exercise routine.** This would ideally include getting up from sitting every hour or two and moving around. Routine contraction of the leg muscles prevents pooling of venous and lymphatic drainage.

- **Avoid wearing tight-fitting clothing, especially around the waist and thighs.** Compression of the lymphatic drainage at these points promotes accumulation of fluid in the fatty tissue of the buttocks, hips, and thighs. Pantyhose may be the biggest culprit here.

- **Avoid sitting and/or crossing the legs for long periods of time.** Get up and move around frequently to improve blood flow and circulation to the lower body. This allows the removal of accumulated toxins from these tissues and improves oxygenation of healthy cells.

- **Consider lymphatic drainage and cellulite massage.** We use the *Lipotherapie* technique in our office with very favorable results. This technique makes use of a therapeutic massage machine, which utilizes a combination of variable suction pressures along with mechanical rolling of the tissue. The massage seems to improve the healthy appearance of the skin as it contours and shapes the cellulitic areas. This procedure is also complementary to weight loss, as it tones loose skin and stimulates blood flow. Although no mechanical device will substitute for healthy habits and skills, Lipothera-pie has turned out to be a resourceful modality when life's pressures preclude a comprehensive cellulite pre-vention program.

- **Practice deep-breathing exercises several times a day.** This practice is a healthy way to stimulate lymphatic flow from the pelvis to the chest where it enters the bloodstream.

- **Perform a gentle brushing of the areas of cellulite on a daily basis.** This is best done with a soft brush using very gentle strokes across the affected areas. Stroking toward the heart stimulates lymphatic drainage in the proper direction.

Cellulite may be viewed as a continuation of the effects of food intolerance. As we have established earlier in this book, food intolerance can make you fat. Now we understand that food intolerance, if not eliminated, will make existing fat deposits even more unsightly. Find out and eliminate your reactive foods.

CHAPTER 12

Fatigue and Food Intolerance

My goodness, is it really that simple, Doctor? After all those years of seeing so many doctors and spending hundreds of dollars on supplements, then, just by not eating my allergenic foods, my fatigue is completely gone.

That comment is from Cheryl, a woman in her mid-30s who had suffered for years with chronic fatigue. In early 1990, she went to see Dr. David Cafarelli at the suggestion of a friend. After years of trying many different therapies to rid her of the constant fatigue that plagued her life, she'd nearly given up hope that any doctor could help her. As soon as she described her medical history to Dr. Cafarelli, he tested her for food intolerance; sure enough, she was sensitive to several foods, including three she was eating nearly every day—tomatoes, potatoes, and eggplant.

Dr. David Cafarelli, a medical practitioner in West Palm Beach for the past 14 years, sees many people with chronic illnesses, including fatigue, who've tried everything and can't get well. Nutritional treatments are a big part of his therapy, including testing for food intolerance using the ALCAT test. "I go by the motto that anything as fundamental as eating is imperative to look at before you move on and get fancy with other tests and treatments," he says. "When a person has food intolerance, which I believe includes nearly everyone, I'm able to find the offending foods right away with this test."

Fatigue: An Early Warning

Fatigue is a common feature of many diseases and illnesses. Evidence implicates food intolerance as a cause of fatigue and even suggests that fatigue may be an "early warning sign" of food intolerance.

Fatigue may be an "early warning sign" of food intolerance.

Dr. Paul Jaconello, a nutritional and preventive medicine specialist in Ontario, Canada, also believes that food is a fundamental part of a complete medical diagnosis, particularly in the area of chronic fatigue. "Certain foods in certain people can trigger a 'biochemical cascade.' Once the body is overloaded, these reactions can manifest as excessive fatigue or they can manifest in any organ of the body, or both." One of his patients, named Jamie, had reached a point of overload while dealing with her mother's death due to lung cancer.

The death was a wakeup call to address her own health, and in her grief she tried to give up smoking. But 38 years of not watching her diet, combined with the stress of her mother's death, overloaded her system; her cholesterol level skyrocketed, and she started gaining weight. A conventional high-carbohydrate diet, prescribed by a dietitian to address Jamie's high cholesterol, left her feeling lethargic, and she started retaining water. Dr. Jaconello suggested that eliminating her food intolerances might help. The ALCAT test showed her intolerant to common foods such as wheat, broccoli, potatoes, grapefruit, and oranges. Not long after removing these foods from her diet, her cholesterol level returned to normal range, her energy level and mental clarity climbed, and the water retention was significantly reduced.

Fatigue may be an "early warning sign" of food intolerance. Cindy, another fatigue sufferer, also decided that something wasn't right after she finally lost weight on a popular diet. The diet left her feeling constantly hungry, fatigued, and cold. The ALCAT test, prescribed by Dr. Richard Bahr, a specialist in environmental medicine in Cincinnati, showed her to be allergic to several foods, including soybeans, zucchini, tomatoes, wheat, and tuna. She said that she ate soybeans, zucchini, and tomatoes often. She strictly followed the prescribed rotation diet—and the tiredness was gone. "I was amazed at how much more energy I had," she said. "When we identify their major food intolerances, patients usually respond rather well," notes Dr. Bahr.

Cheryl, Jamie, and Cindy's stories are not unusual. Like so many others with serious medical conditions, many people have been cured of fatigue—including low energy and chronic fatigue syndrome—by eliminating the foods to which they showed intolerance. Normally, people experience fatigue after they've exerted a great deal of energy. However, if their tiredness is not related to any particular exertion on their part, is unrelieved by rest or sleep, and is frequently worse in the morning, many health practitioners believe it is probably associated in some way with food and/or chemical sensitivities. Persistent fatigue, although not necessarily life-threatening, can be a debilitating, life-wrecking medical condition, severely limiting a person's potential, both personally and professionally. Yet it is widespread and appears, like many medical conditions caused by food intolerance, to be growing.

Most experts find fatigue so common that putting a number on how many people suffer from excessive tiredness is impossible. According to a *Health* magazine report (October 1995), "One in four Americans have fatigue lasting longer than two weeks, often beyond six months." In a May 14, 1979, issue of *U.S. News and World Report*, Dr. John E. Bulette, a psychiatrist at the Medical College of Pennsylvania, stated that 50 percent of all patients admitted to general hospitals in the United States list fatigue as a major complaint. According to Dr. Theron Randolph, in *An Alternative Approach to Allergies* (1982, reprinted 1990), "One of the most commonly occurring symptoms in medicine, and especially in the histories of allergy patients, is chronic fatigue. Although fatigue may be the only manifestation of their problem, it more commonly exists in conjunction with other manifestations."

Whereas many people are like Cheryl, Jamie, and Cindy, for whom fatigue is the dominant symptom, another category of patients exists for whom fatigue is a secondary symptom that accompanies a major symptom, and who can also be helped by addressing food allergy. In fact it's not unusual for patients who have been evaluated with the ALCAT test for a number of symptoms, such as obesity, irritable bowel, or migraines, and who have eliminated the foods they do not tolerate, to remark, "I have so much more energy!"

Christine, for example, was so "bone weary" in 1990 that she couldn't put one foot in front of the other, even though she slept all night long. For several months before the onset of her severe fatigue, her health had been deteriorating. In particular, she was experiencing increasingly severe chest pains and heart palpitations, and she had muscle aches in her arms. Finally, her condition landed her in the hospital. While there, she became even more tired and achy. Two days after she returned home, she was back in the hospital with severe chest pains and a rash that had developed all over her body. Her doctors were mystified by her condition; try as they might, they couldn't find the source of her mounting problems.

When she left the hospital for the second time, she immediately made an appointment with Dr. Barbara Solomon, an internal medicine physician who specializes in alternative therapies in Maryland. Dr. Solomon had successfully treated Christine's husband for a chronic, debilitating skin rash by locating his food intolerances. Dr. Solomon had an ALCAT test completed on Christine. As soon as Christine stopped eating the foods she does not tolerate, she felt better. "It was unbelievable. From the very day I stopped eating my untolerated foods I started getting better. The tiredness lifted, the chest pains subsided, and the rash disappeared. My primary care physician couldn't believe how fast I improved. Also, I learned that the reason I had felt so much worse in the hospital was the food they fed me, like chicken, potatoes, and green beans, all of which I am highly reactive to."

Few people respond as quickly as Christine did, but her story dramatically illustrates the fact that traditional medical practices rarely recognize food intolerance, even when it's right under their noses, as it was when Christine was in the hospital. I have been impressed with the number of patients in my own practice who relate how much more energetic they feel after the first week away from their reactive foods.

Oralia was at her wits' end. She was 35 years old, unemployed, and living with her mother because she could not hold a job due to her constant fatigue, gastrointestinal problems, memory loss, and allergies. She had seen a conventional gastroenterologist and had been subjected to barium swallows, barium enemas, endoscopes, colonoscopes, and everything else the doctor could think of doing for her constant belching, flatulence, and intestinal bloating. After all the tests came back negative for any specific disease, the doctor told her that there was nothing that could be done for her except for maybe putting her on some antacid medications.

She finally went to see Dr. David M. Brady, a nutrition-oriented functional medicine practitioner at the University of Bridgeport in Connecticut. He explored interrelationships among her myriad of symptoms. ALCAT testing on her revealed that she had a significant intolerance to corn and dairy, two main components of her Mexican-influenced diet. By avoiding these foods and engaging in other therapies to heal her injured intestinal lining, she recovered rapidly, was able to find and hold a job, and ultimately was able to move out on her own and become a productive member of society again. Like many others, she was absolutely amazed that something as simple as removing some of the foods that she was regularly eating could make such a profound influence on her health and indeed her entire life.

More Common Than You'd Think

Even though it's so common, fatigue almost seems to not be considered a serious medical condition by the general medical community. Even the debilitating disease known as chronic fatigue syndrome gets short shrift from most doctors. An article in *Newsweek* in April 1996 reported that "There is no question the health establishment has erred on the side of complacency." As a result, many people with hidden food allergies that manifest as fatigue, and with other symptoms, go to doctor after doctor seeking relief.

Denise, for example, is the kind of patient whom doctors derogatorily refer to as hypochondriacs or as having "thick file syndrome" because they go to doctors so often complaining about so many different symptoms. Denise went from one doctor to another for nine years complaining of fatigue, sore muscles, a painful knot in her shoulder, depression, sinus problems, weight gain, and insomnia. Although she would insist something was wrong with her, the doctors would make comments such as "You're just stressed because you're a busy mom" or the classic "It's all in your head." When she was 56 pounds overweight, one doctor prescribed diet pills. "I had more energy, but they sped me up so much that I dumped them in the toilet. The last thing I needed, on top of everything else, was to become addicted to drugs."

She never got any relief from any of her symptoms until she went to see Dr. Anthony Ferro in West Chester, Pennsylvania. He suspected food intolerance and ordered an ALCAT test. Denise was intolerant to a long list of foods, including wheat, potatoes, sugar, dairy products, and several vegetables. She'd been eating these foods nearly every day as prescribed by various weight loss diets. By modifying her diet she immediately lost weight and the fatigue lifted, as did all her other symptoms. "I had felt like I was on the road to death, spinning out of control. I was surprised to find that I had any food allergies, let alone so many. I was very pleased to find the solution as simple as food allergies, because if I'd stayed on a low-calorie diet and prescription drugs I would be much worse off today."

Many people like Denise feel that their lives were literally rescued by finding out that allergenic foods were making them sick and tired. A popular opera singer in Denmark was living a celebrity's pampered lifestyle, including eating the best food and drinking the best wine that money could buy, until the day he collapsed on stage. Just prior to his collapse, the Royal Opera House was being renovated and dust was everywhere. Suddenly, one night while performing, his throat closed, his eyes burned, and he became so tired he had to be carried off the stage. After that episode he couldn't return to the stage, due to both his fear and to his extreme exhaustion.

Terrified for his health and his career, he traveled to the United States to see one of the leading allergy experts; ironically, it wasn't until he returned to Denmark and was referred to Dr. Lene Høj, a Danish allergist in Copenhagen, that he got relief. She tested him for food and chemical allergies and found several of both, including calves' liver, to which he was so reactive that it was "pure poison" for him. He went on a strict diet and had his home cleared of all chemicals. He became a discriminating eater at parties and brought his own sulfite-free wine when socializing. Within a short time he was able to return to the stage.

The opera singer's experience is one of many classic stories that help confirm the belief of many environmental and preventive health physicians—that one reason a food intolerance manifests is because the body reaches a state of overload. This performer had been eating all the wrong foods, drinking the wrong beverages, and living with toxins that were depressing his body's immune system. His daily exposure to a new allergen—dust mites—was the proverbial straw that broke the camel's back, and he could no longer continue taxing his system with the toxins in certain foods and chemicals.

Trail Benedict believes that his and his father's systems were overloaded from working in the family's chemical laboratory business, where they handled many pesticides. Both suffered from extreme fatigue—Trail to the point that he was falling asleep while driving to work, despite getting a good night's sleep every night. His family switched to the nutritional supplement business in the early 1980s, but none of the supplements they sold to others for improving health gave them more energy. Finally, Trail and his father learned about the ALCAT test. Once they eliminated their allergenic foods, both had more energy than they'd had in years. Trail also lost 20 pounds he'd wanted to shed. "Eliminating our allergenic foods had a dramatic effect on our health. I knew I had allergies but I couldn't pinpoint them. The ALCAT identified them for me."

Further Evidence Links Food to Fatigue

Patient success stories are not the only proof that food intolerance can be the culprit in fatigue and low energy. Many of the researchers, including prominent professionals in the field of food intolerance, consistently find a strong link between food allergies and fatigue. As early as 1946, Dr. Theron Randolph published studies on allergy as a causative factor in fatigue and weakness. In 1950, Dr. Albert Rowe published a paper on allergic toxemia and fatigue. And in 1954, Dr. Frederic Speer published a study on fatigue and its relationship to food allergy. Dr. William Crook in 1961 also listed fatigue as one of the systemic manifestations due to allergy in children.

Current research studies on the ALCAT test also show that addressing food intolerance does lead to improvement in people's fatigue symptoms. One study was conducted by Dr. Barbara Solomon to determine whether the ALCAT test was a valuable technique for physicians treating environmental illness. She studied a group of 172 patients seen in her primary-care internal medicine practice for a wide range of symptoms, including fatigue, depression, migraines, gastrointestinal problems, arthritis, asthma, obesity, and eczema. Dr. Solomon reported that of the 97 cases of tension fatigue syndrome, 60 percent of the patients improved just from removing their allergenic foods from their diets. "These patients were among a category of patients who come to me as a last resort. They never suspected that foods trigger their symptoms."

One study found that the ALCAT test has a truly predictable capacity for detecting food sensitivity. Dr. Peter Fell, a clinical pharmacologist who had been the medical director of a major pharmaceutical company but later took up the practice of allergy, and Dr. Jonathan Brostoff, from the Department of Immunology at the University College and Middlesex Hospital Medicine School, found that all the females in the study, aged 20 to 45, who presented with fatigue syndrome showed improvement by eliminating allergenic foods.

In a study on the relationship of food intolerance to weight loss, body composition, and self-reported disease symptoms conducted in 1994 at the Columbia/HCA Medical Center's Sports Medicine and Performance Center in Houston, lead investigator Gilbert Kaats, Ph.D., found a marked improvement in chronic tiredness, tension fatigue syndrome, lack of energy, and insomnia when sufferers eliminated their intolerant foods. Although both the experimental group and control group (50 participants each) initially reported the same degree of chronic tiredness, the people on an individualized ALCAT diet for four weeks reported that their tiredness had improved by 50 percent. People who followed diets of their own choosing for four weeks reported no change in their chronic tiredness.

The people following an ALCAT diet, however, reported a 67 percent improvement. With the symptom "lack of energy," the ALCAT dieters reported just over 50 percent improvement, whereas the non-ALCAT dieters reported only about 10 percent improvement. With insomnia, the ALCAT dieters reported nearly 66 percent improvement at the end of the study, whereas the control group reported barely 5 percent improvement. "In all four categories these findings are highly statistically significant," explains Dr. Kaats, director of the Health and Medical Research Foundation, an independent research organization in San Antonio, Texas. "The chance of these results occurring at random is very slim. In other words, if you repeated the study 1,000 times, 999 times you would get the same scores for tension fatigue syndrome, and you would get the same scores 996 times for chronic tiredness and insomnia. This is a good indication that the results are not due to random chance."

Other doctors have also found success treating patients with fatigue by eliminating their sensitive foods. "Chronic fatigue patients often have underlying food sensitivities," says Dr. Jaconello. Dr. Ronald Lesko is well known in the area of metabolic problems, allergies, and chronic fatigue, and treats many patients from all over the United States. He tests the majority of them for food intolerance using the ALCAT test and finds the test helpful in diagnosing the cause of symptoms and in designing a dietetic program to treat the fatigue. Dr. Stephen Smith, of Richland, Washington, says, "I treat people with chronic fatigue, and we do have success."

Even with scientific studies, patients' personal experiences, and physicians' success stories, the fact that fatigue (including chronic fatigue syndrome) can be alleviated by eliminating intolerant foods from a person's diet is not generally accepted by the medical community. But physicians who accept food intolerance believe, like Dr. Theron Randolph, that fatigue may be the most characteristic part of food and chemical susceptibility. They believe that if no obvious medical condition, such as heart problems, chronic infection, or cancer exists, food or chemical allergy should definitely be suspected. "The majority of allergic individuals with the fatigue syndrome have been previously diagnosed as 'neurotics,'" notes Dr. Randolph, due to physicians' typical separation of mental and physical problems. But he found that chemicals in the environment are slowly poisoning them, as their reactions to commonly eaten foods indicate. It's no wonder that patients who are chronically fatigued develop mental symptoms as well. Who wouldn't be upset if they were too exhausted to live their lives and fulfill their responsibilities?

Why So Tired?

Professor Jonathan Brostoff points out in *The Complete Guide to Food Allergy and Intolerance* (1992) that excessive tiredness can be caused by many infectious diseases, by anemia, or by an underactive thyroid gland, which can also be brought on by food intolerance. "Fatigue is very often reported as a symptom of food intolerance, especially in connection with migraines and irritable bowel syndrome. Early-morning tiredness is the most frequent problem. Looking back over case histories, it seems that fatigue may be an early warning sign as food intolerance develops." How foods might produce fatigue is not known. But Professor Brostoff suggests that exorphines (peptides very similar to endorphins, which are natural opioids that help turn off pain in our bodies) may play a part, or fatigue may be a side effect of some generalized immune reaction, as is suspected in postviral syndrome.

In a great number of cases, fatigue persists following a viral infection, and this is now known as postviral syndrome or chronic fatigue syndrome. Because it has received so much press, chronic fatigue syndrome is a well-known, often misdiagnosed condition. Although many people are chronically tired, true chronic fatigue syndrome is characterized by debilitating tiredness for over six months. It is accompanied by a long list of symptoms, including cognitive function problems, visual disturbances, psychological problems, shortness of breath, dizziness and balance problems, sensitivity to extreme temperatures, and chest pains, according to the Chronic Fatigue and Immune Dysfunction Syndrome Association of America (CFIDSAA).

A great deal of study has been done on chronic fatigue syndrome—which is believed to affect 4 to 10 out of every 100,000 adults—with few, if any, conclusive answers. Beginning in the early 1990s, a growing number of researchers concluded that chronic fatigue is a serious, albeit mysterious, medical problem. Some believe it's caused by a virus, because many people come down with the syndrome soon after a flulike illness. When you get an infection, you produce proteins called cytokines, which facilitate communication between and activate certain white blood cells, which then devour bacteria and other invaders. In addition to killing the invaders, cytokines also lay you low, and their effects can persist for some time.

Other sufferers get chronic fatigue after a psychological trauma, or a period of intense work, suggesting that stress hormones may cause it. Those who treat it as a real disease generally agree on a few basic ideas. One theory is that chronic fatigue syndrome results from a dysfunction of the immune system. A virus, stress, or another trauma somehow jumpstarts the immune system, which then remains activated instead of gearing down as it would after an infection. As a result, a number of immune factors (some of which cause fatigue) remain indefinitely in high concentrations in the blood.

According to the CFIDSAA in 1997, "The exact nature of this dysfunction is not well defined, . . . but it can generally be viewed as an up-regulated or overactive state. Ironically, there is also evidence of some immune suppression. For example, in many patients there are functional deficiencies in natural killer cells (an important component of the immune system responsible for fighting viruses)." In other words, these patients have a compromised immune system, which is weak and at the same time hyperactive. This paradox is not uncommon. Often when an organ has to work overtime, because of some primary deficiency, it becomes enlarged. For example, the pancreas becomes enlarged when, in order to aid digestion, it is required to produce extra enzymes to compensate for the consumption of enzyme-deficient foods.

This thinking correlates with Brostoff's research in the area of fatigue and the immune system. He points out that all lymphocytes produce small messenger molecules, known as lymphokines, to communicate with each other. One important messenger molecule is interferon, whose main job is to combat viral infections. Interferon makes cells resistant to virus, but it also produces a long list of side effects such as severe fatigue, dizziness, joint pain, and headaches—symptoms remarkably similar to those of chronic fatigue syndrome. Because most cases seem to follow a viral infection of some sort, the parallel with the side effects of interferon suggests that "the immune system has overreacted to a viral infection and is continuing to produce excessive amounts of interferon. If this is the case (and there is no definitive proof that it is), then interferon might also play a role in food intolerance. Perhaps some unknown immune reaction to food stimulates the body to produce interferon, or other lymphokines, in damaging amounts. It is interesting that many chronic fatigue sufferers have been greatly helped by an elimination diet—it would seem that reactions to food are contributing to their symptoms."

Energetic Again

If this theory can be proven, it would explain Cleason's experience with chronic fatigue syndrome (see chapter 1). In December 1986, Cleason developed a bad flu. It lingered longer than usual and finally seemed to resolve. Then in March he got another flu, after which he just couldn't wake up. Constant headaches and diarrhea accompanied his daily fatigue. He dragged himself out of bed and pushed himself to go to work. Soon he started missing work. By September, the fatigue had taken its full toll and he stopped working altogether.

For all those months he saw one doctor after another with no relief. He got to the point that he lost confidence in the doctors' ability to help him. But with eight children and a wife to support, he had to try something. Finally, his wife encouraged him to have an ALCAT test. Two of their children, one of whom was hyperactive and one who had gastrointestinal problems, had been successfully treated for food sensitivities. Cleason was tested for 100 foods, and for mold and pollen allergies. He showed a long list of sensitivities. As soon as he stopped eating his reactive foods, he was 75 percent improved. By dealing with his mold and pollen allergies, he was able to return to his former self.

Although the "why" of chronic fatigue may be longer in coming, it's enough for the people like Christine, Denise, Trail, and Cleason, who have already found relief from their tiredness, to know that something as simple as removing their sensitive foods allowed them to return to normal lives.

In Summary

As Dr. David M. Brady, chair of the department of clinical sciences at the University of Bridgeport Colleges of Chiropractic and Naturopathic Medicine, and published expert on fatigue-related disorders, states,

> In any patient with long-standing fatigue, food, chemical, and substance intolerance must be included in the patient's assessment. Unfortunately, many busy physicians today do not even adequately assess the well-known and accepted reasons for fatigue, such as anemia, infection, hypothyroidism, and serious internal diseases like cancer, in the patients who present to them complaining of being constantly tired. Screening for these disorders is as simple as ordering a few relatively inexpensive and routine blood tests. However, in today's busy managed care environments the patient is more likely to be immediately labeled with a trendy "catch-all" or "wastebasket" diagnosis such as chronic fatigue syndrome or fibromyalgia and put on anti-depressant medications, as if their problems are all in their heads. Not that those disorders, such as chronic fatigue and fibromyalgia, do not exist, but many of the patients given those diagnoses do not even have the routine potential reasons for their problems ruled out. If these well accepted tests are not even being done, how can the patient expect the general physician to consider a novel testing procedure like the ALCAT test? In our center, we make sure to rule out these common medical disorders, as well as a host of other more subtle "functional" problems such as certain types of thyroid and adrenal gland dysfunctions that are not commonly detected on standard laboratory studies, as well as toxicity, and intestinal disorders. We also train our student physicians to actually listen to the patient's story, and to consider lifestyle issues such as stress, diet, and activity level in assessing the reason for the patient's problem. For instance, it must be appreciated that intolerance to a food that we commonly eat can cause an ongoing inflammatory reaction on the lining of the intestines, which can result in that lining becoming unhealthy and "leaky." In other words, it does not keep certain substances from being absorbed into our blood stream as it should, such as partially undigested food proteins and large toxins, which result in an upregulated immune response. This flood

of "bad" material into the blood stream overburdens the liver's ability to detoxify these substances, thereby creating a great deal of oxidative stress in the body. Ultimately, this oxidative stress has been known to contribute to the genesis of a multitude of degenerative disorders, such as heart disease and cancer. However, that stress has an even more frequent effect on the mitochondria, which are the energy-producing parts of our cells. The eventual result is fatigue, brain-fog, degenerative disease, and a never-ending cycle of more and more allergy and intolerance. For this reason, we utilize the ALCAT test as an invaluable tool in directing our fatigued patients back to a full and vital life by detecting what they are intolerant to and coaching them in the avoidance of those substances. After dozens of trips from specialists to specialists for these patients without a clean diagnosis or cure, it is often just that simple.

So it is seen, as with many common problems, food and chemical intolerance play a significant role in symptoms of fatigue.

CHAPTER 13

Migraine and Food Intolerance

I used to have severe migraines two or three times a week," explains Sylvia. "During those attacks I became nauseous and tired. If I didn't have the chance to lie down, I had to take two or three very strong pain relievers to survive the day. On the weekends, I'd spend one or both days in bed. Now that I am no longer eating my intolerant foods, my migraines are completely gone. I'm so grateful to finally have relief and to live a normal life again."

This is one of many letters that thankful patients have written to Mr. Just Hintz, manager of a laboratory in Germany where doctors process their patients' ALCAT blood tests. And the writer is just one of many grateful migraine sufferers around the world who finally found relief—amid the various notions of how to treat migraines—after learning which foods their bodies tolerate, and by avoiding those foods. "We've found that most times, with migraines, patients improve," notes Hintz.

I've Got a Headache

Only a migraine sufferer can understand the excruciating, throbbing pain of this condition which, at its worse, can land a sufferer in bed for an occasional day or incapacitate them for several days each week. These debilitating headaches are often accompanied by vision sensitivities (even temporary blindness), nausea, shaking, vomiting, fatigue, depression, skin problems, and irritable bowel, all symptoms that compound the suffering. Statistically, each year in the United States, headaches cripple more people than motorcycle accidents, car collisions, and industrial accidents combined. Over 45 million Americans get chronic, recurring headaches, and that number increases every year. Of this number, 16 to 18 million suffer from migraines, and 70 percent of all migraine sufferers are women.

These chronic, recurring headaches are severe enough to cause those in pain to seek medical attention and, in some cases, prevent them from maintaining full-time employment. According to the National Headache Foundation, by 1995 headaches cost industry a $50 billion loss due to absenteeism and medical expenses, and migraines caused sufferers to lose more than 157 million workdays. In excess of $4 billion is spent annually on over-the-counter pain relievers for headaches, many of which are ineffective.

In the United Kingdom, migraine sufferers comprise the largest group attending neurological clinics—up to one-third of all patients in some centers. Some estimates have placed the incidence of migraine in the population as high as 30 percent. In that country, more working days are lost due to headache than through any other single category of complaint. When migraineurs try to work with a headache, they are less efficient. And many feel they cannot plan their work and social lives for fear of being devastated by a headache.

Of the several types of headaches, most fall into one of three basic categories: tension-type headaches that bring an ache in the area where the muscles of the head and neck meet; vascular headaches, which include migraines, toxic, and cluster headaches; and organically caused headaches from tumors, infections, and disease. Many popular treatments are available—including prescription and over-the-counter medications, vertebra realignment, and psychotherapy—yet the excruciating head pain still continues for millions. Often sufferers search their whole lives for help, willing to try anything that even remotely claims to be a cure. Many choose to suffer the dangerous side effects of drugs, including constricted blood vessels around the heart as well as in the brain, rather than endure a migraine's wrath.

Some headache sufferers, however, have found the simple, drug-free solution—treatment for food intolerance. Thousands of patients and dozens of research studies show that identifying and eliminating their intolerant foods is a viable solution for many. How removing food (and chemical) intolerances works to alleviate migraines is not clear. Up to now, the cause of headaches has been attributed to hormonal imbalance, genetic predisposition, chronic tension, and emotional issues, with some foods cited as the triggers. However, physicians who recognize food intolerance as a cause of headaches agree that medical professionals who ignore food allergy cannot get the whole picture. As Dr. Richard Bahr, an environmental medicine specialist in Cincinnati, puts it: "We know that migraines are a food problem until you can prove otherwise. They are not all food-related, but the greater percent are."

"A large portion of head pain, including even the worst forms of migraine, are simply due to allergic reactions," writes Dr. Theron Randolph in *An Alternative*

Approach to Allergies. This simple fact has been the answer to many migraineurs' prayers. For example, Ruth, one of Dr. Ivonne Torre-Coya's migraine patients, found out through the ALCAT Test that she was intolerant to coffee and grapes, both of which she consumed frequently. "When she cut them out of her diet, the effect was incredible. Her headaches disappeared," explains Carmen, assistant to Dr. Torre-Coya, a physician and allergy specialist in Miami. "She was really happy, and feeling great."

Another grateful German patient who wrote to Mr. Hintz had this to say: "I took the ALCAT Test for my chronic sinus allergy problem, and after removing my allergenic foods, particularly wheat, there was a nice side effect—I don't have my migraines anymore, which I got quite often before."

Identifying "Trigger" Foods

It's common to hear that certain foods trigger migraines—for example, aged cheese, chocolate, and red wine are often implicated. But you'll never hear popular medical focus on lamb, milk, or wheat. Yet those are the foods that caused Tom, Sharon, and Barbara to suffer from excruciating headaches and migraines, no matter which of the commonly accepted headache-trigger foods they eliminated from their diets. Dr. Anthony Ferro in Palm Beach, who has successfully treated many patients with migraine, noted: "I have one patient, Tom, who gets a migraine whenever he eats wheat."

Sharon, a 52-year-old public relations consultant, is in generally good health except for severe migraines. For years she managed her migraines, which only occurred every once in awhile, by taking over-the-counter pain medications. Then, out of the blue, the migraines picked up in frequency and intensity; at least once a week she'd be way-laid by stabbing pain around the eyes and nausea that persisted for two hours. "I prefer not to take a lot of medications. But the increasingly severe headaches were starting to cut into my lifestyle. As a public relations consultant, I have a very active social life, and you don't exactly feel like going out dancing when you have a migraine."

Finally tested with the ALCAT Test at the suggestion of a business acquaintance, Sharon was surprised to learn that she was allergic to two of her favorite foods—lamb and chocolate—in addition to tomatoes, salmon, wheat, and dairy products, all of which she ate frequently. Looking back, she realized that her headaches had picked up in intensity when she started eating regularly at a new Mediterranean restaurant near her office. "I wasn't pleased to find out that I was reactive to foods I liked, so I decided to test the test. I ate lamb one day for lunch, and sure enough, an hour later I developed a migraine headache. I realized that there's a lot of validity here. With migraines, you don't want to test too much. But as per my doctor's recommendations, I did test it again a few months later and got another migraine within an hour or two of eating lamb. That was enough testing for me. Now I choose another dish at my favorite restaurant."

Dr. Barbara Solomon in Baltimore became interested in allergy in the mid-1960s when, as an internal medicine resident, she slowly started getting migraines. First she'd get one every three months, then monthly. Before long she was experiencing a migraine every week, then three times a week, until finally she had a constant migraine, including vomiting. This went on for a year until she could no longer stand the agonizing pain. Instinctively, she decided to try changing her diet. Because beef and milk were the main two foods in her busy life as a medical resident, she tried eliminating them. Dr. Solomon recalls:

I was amazed when the migraines went away. At the time, I didn't know about the research on food intolerance and headaches. But I thought: I'm not unique; there are other people with headaches and it's probably food related. If changing my diet worked for me, it might work for other people.

The first headache patient I tried this theory on ate nothing but cheese and wheat. So I advised him to cut both out of his diet, and I hit it right. When he didn't eat the foods, the headaches went away; when he ate them again, the headaches came back. I kept doing this with headache patients, and they kept getting better.

So every time I had a headache patient, I'd have them keep a food diary for a few weeks, then I'd advise them to give up the foods they ate the most frequently. Most of them got better. I'd challenge the result by having them add the foods back into their diets, and invariably they would get sick again. Then I decided that I had to have a test that could quickly tell me exactly to which foods my patients were intolerant. For nearly 20 years I used the only food intolerance testing method available at the time. But in the past 10 years I've been using the ALCAT Test. It's a much more convenient and efficient test.

Migraine and Intolerance:
Research Confirms the Connection

Dr. Solomon has since conducted research on the ALCAT Test to determine its effectiveness as a guide and barometer in the therapy of environmental and food sensitivities. Her study not only confirmed that the ALCAT Test is a valuable guide in quickly identifying a person's food, mold, and chemical allergies, but it also showed that several conditions, including migraines, can be improved by addressing food intolerance. "The traditional medical community says that classic migraine is not food allergy, but in my experience it is," says Dr. Solomon.

Her study included 71 patients with headaches. Of the nine patients with classic migraine (which includes visual disturbances such as flashing lights and split vision), 82 percent showed improvement after eliminating the foods to which they tested reactive. Of the 39 patients with common migraine (which includes no visual disturbances), 62 percent showed improvement. And of the 23 patients with sinus headaches, 58 percent showed improvement. "My study showed that eliminating food intolerances is effective in clearing a person's migraine 82 percent of the time, and 82 percent is pretty good."

In two studies they conducted on migraines and food intolerance using the ALCAT Test, Drs. Fell and Brostoff found excellent results for headache and migraine sufferers. In the first study, conducted in 1988, 80 patients with a variety of conditions including migraine were observed. Drs. Fell and Brostoff showed that this simple blood test, as opposed to guesswork, enabled them to identify patients' food intolerance, and the patients who stopped eating the sensitive foods showed clear-cut improvement of migraines, while the patients who continued to eat their allergic foods showed "disastrous results." In a second study conducted in 1990, 14 of 18 patients with migraines got better. During the 12-month study, these patients' improvement was measured by scoring all four target symptoms—aura, headache, nausea, and vomiting. All maintained their success. "Interestingly, several of the patients said that although an aura developed, there was a failure of the full-blown syndrome to develop with headache, nausea, and vomiting," explains Brostoff.

A study on the relationship of food intolerance to weight loss, body composition, and self-reported disease symptoms was conducted in 1995 at the Columbia/HCA Medical Center's Sports Medicine and Performance Center in Houston and Baylor Medical College Sports Medicine and Performance Institute. Lead investigator Gilbert Kaats, Ph.D., director of the Health and Medical Research Foundation, an independent research organization in San Antonio, found that people on an ALCAT diet who reported suffering from migraines improved by 50 percent within four weeks. Migraine sufferers who followed diets of their own choosing said that their head pain had only improved by about 25 percent at the end of the four-week study.

The idea that allergenic foods can cause headaches is not new. Many researchers have discovered a relationship between allergy and migraines. As far back as 1905, the Australian medical pioneer Dr. Francis Hare reported that head pain could be the result of eating incompatible foods. In 1927, two prominent American allergists, Drs. Albert H. Rowe and Warren T. Vaughn, both published articles implicating specific foods as the cause of allergic headaches.

In a study in 1930, Dr. Rowe again found migraines to be related to food allergy. In 1934, Dr. A. Andresen reported that migraine was an allergic phenomenon. In 1979, Dr. C. G. Grant reported that diet led to freedom from migraine attacks in 51 of 60 patients, while the other nine patients experienced a reduction in headache frequency. In 1985, Dr. Lyndon Mansfield, president of the American In Vitro Allergy and Immunology Society and an allergy specialist in private practice in El Paso, Texas, published a study on food allergy and the adult migraine that showed a clear relationship between migraines and allergic disease. With guesswork alone to identify causative foods, Dr. Mansfield observed that 6 out of 43 patients became headache-free, and 13 subjects experienced 66 percent or greater reduction in headache frequency.

In 1935, Dr. Theron Randolph wrote a medical paper entitled "Allergy in Migraine-like Headaches," based on his work while at the University of Michigan Medical School. In this paper, he observed that two-thirds of the migraine patients at the University Hospital in Ann Arbor obtained relief from headaches by eliminating various foods from their diets. In 1989, he wrote, "These results are certainly better than those achieved by conventional medicine. There is no need for a person to suffer for years on end with persistent headaches when the cause of these disorders can often be identified and relieved by eliminating certain common substances from the environment. Today, however, even better results can be achieved through the diagnosis of chemical susceptibility and of some common food allergies, which had not then been identified." He notes that there is no mass-applicable shortcut to finding intolerant foods and controlling headaches. What affects one patient does not trouble the next. Individual testing using the ALCAT Test is needed.

Pain, Pain, Go Away: Children and Migraines

Adults are not the only ones to suffer from headaches and migraines; children do as well. Headaches in children are thought to be genetically inherited from parents who have migraines. Studies show that 70 to 80 percent of migraines have a hereditary influence. If both parents have them, children have a 75 percent chance of having migraines as well. When one parent suffers from migraines, the child will have a 50 percent chance of being afflicted. Dr. Joseph Egger, who works at the Childrens' Hospital in

Munich, Germany, posed the question "Is Migraine Food Allergy?" in a study of children's headaches published in a 1983 issue of *The Lancet.* He found that when 78 of 88 children who experienced headaches at least once a week eliminated certain foods from their diets, they completely recovered from the migraines, as well as associated symptoms like abdominal pain, behavior disorders, asthma, and eczema.

Many parents have been greatly relieved to find a simple, noninvasive, nonmedicating solution to their children's debilitating headaches.

This study also resulted in three interesting conclusions: (1) offending foods were most often unsuspected and often the person's favorite foods; (2) although 17 of the 88 subjects were allergic to only one food, the rest were allergic to a number of foods; and (3) one child had to eliminate 24 foods before getting relief from migraines. Traditional allergy tests available at the time—skin tests and RAST (radioallergosorbent test, a laboratory test specific for IgE antibodies)—were of no value in detecting food intolerances.

Many parents have been greatly relieved to find a simple, noninvasive, nonmedicating solution to their children's debilitating headaches. At the suggestion of Dr. John Gerrard, her children's physician and an expert in allergy and immunology in Saskatchewan, Canada, Shirley removed sweets, chocolate, cola, and dairy products from her 12-year-old son Bruce's diet. His headaches went away.

Jackie's son Trent began having headaches and showing signs of hyperactivity at three years old. At the suggestion of her doctor, Jackie had Trent tested at age four using the ALCAT Test. While his hyperactivity rapidly improved by eliminating the intolerant foods, his migraines took a couple months to completely disappear. "I wasn't as concerned about the hyperactivity as I was about the migraines," explains Jackie. "They were frightening when he got then. He'd have no motor skills for nearly two hours. I don't like to give my child medications. And although it's not easy to feed a young child food they like, if I can alter his diet that is definitely the lesser of two evils." Consistent with the research on the hereditary nature of migraines, Jackie says that she herself had developed migraines while she was pregnant.

Lorraine says that when her children's fifth doctor, Dr. Constantine Kotsanis, a pediatrician in Dallas, suggested food and chemical allergies as an answer to her six-year-old son's attention-deficit-hyperactivity disorder, her four-year-old daughter's autism, and both children's accompanying headaches, she "didn't know what to think. No doctor had ever said anything about allergy being the problem before." Dr. Kotsanis has successfully treated many children with ADHD and other conditions by uncovering their food intolerances using the ALCAT Test. Lorraine's daughter had to eliminate corn, tomato, tuna, shrimp, and blue dye, and avoid some specific molds. Her son had to eliminate chicken, sugar, broccoli, sulfites, and red dye, and avoid most molds.

Like many children, Lorraine's kids responded well to dietary changes. "I was so relieved to find a solution to the migraines. My daughter's were so painful she would bang herself on the head. It seemed like she was always in pain, and it was running me ragged. Now, she no longer bangs herself on the head and her grouchiness and stomachaches are gone. What's more, she is much more receptive to learning than ever before. But if she eats corn or tomatoes, she'll start flying around the room. My six-year-old son had always complained about tummy-ache and headache after eating and now his pain is gone." She says by changing her children's diets, her headaches have gone away, too.

Virginia wishes that doctors had diagnosed her food intolerances when she was a child. If they had, it would have saved her years of pain. As a child Virginia loved cookies and candy as much as the next child and she ate them as often as she could. But she had something her playmates didn't have—severe headaches. Her parents took her to several doctors, "none of whom ever mentioned food allergy being a possible cause to my headaches," Virginia says. Finally, in her teen and college years, her headaches disappeared and she thought she was free from the excruciating pain. Then as a teacher and young mother raising three children, the headaches came back with a vengeance as full-blown migraines, landing her in bed, heavily medicated, at least once a week.

Virginia went to Dr. Anthony Ferro in West Chester, Pennsylvania, for her headaches after the doctor had successfully cured her son's sinus problem. Dr. Ferro ran an ALCAT Test and found her intolerant to several foods, including chocolate, yeast, sugar, eggplant, and green peppers. "Chocolate is totally out," she says. "It gives me such a bad headache, I can't ever eat it. I don't indulge in yeast and sugar much at all. I can have a little bit of green pepper, eggplant, and other nightshade vegetables, but if I ate them every day I'd be in bad shape. Looking back, I realize that during the time I was headache-free, in my teens and during college, was a period when I didn't eat desserts very often."

Virginia went on a bland diet, including completely eliminating her intolerant foods, for six months at the beginning of her therapy to rid her body of the antibiotics she'd been taking to fight her annual bouts of strep throat. While on the bland diet she didn't have a single headache. Since she's been off the bland diet, she has had a few headaches, but nothing like before. She attributes her current headaches to the fact that she is not especially strict with her diet:

"If I do eat desert, I try to eat one with less sugar. I can't even overdo on honey and fruit. I can only have one piece of bread a day because of yeast. I feel really healthy these days. I've only had one bad cold that required antibiotics. I am really grateful to find a solution to controlling the pain, lethargy, and irritability, because the migraines were becoming a definite problem." Like a lot of patients who eliminated foods for symptoms unrelated to weight, Virginia also lost an extra ten pounds she'd been carrying.

The Anatomy of a Migraine

The physical process and cause of headaches and migraines are not yet clearly understood. Current thinking suggests that the aura, or warning associated with migraine (such as vision problems), is due to a narrowing or constriction of the blood vessels supplying the brain and its surrounding tissues, thereby reducing the blood flow to the areas. Following the constriction phase, the blood vessels are then believed to dilate more than normal. The typical pounding headache and migraine is associated with the swelling of the blood vessels surrounding the brain.

Another part of this stage is inflammation caused by the clumping of certain blood cells, the platelets, during an attack. These platelets are tiny cell-type structures in the blood whose main function is to help the blood clot around a wound. During clotting the platelets clump together and release the natural brain neurotransmitter serotonin, which makes the blood vessels constrict to help reduce blood loss. During a migraine attack, the platelets clump together and release large amounts of serotonin when it is not needed. The serotonin makes the blood vessels constrict and so reduces the blood flow to the brain.

The body has control mechanisms that counteract the effect of the serotonin, but these may cause a violent swing in the opposite direction when they come into play. Interestingly, the eicosanoids PGE-2 and PGI-1 are both potent vasodilators. PGE-2 is found in areas of inflammation and is synthesized by platelets, while PGI-1 is synthesized by the blood vessel lining or endothelium and is an antagonist of platelet clumping. The increased production of these eicosanoids in response to the inflammation and platelet clumping associated with a food sensitivity reaction may partially explain many migraine headache reactions. The blood vessels in the brain open up too much, which brings on the throbbing pain that is a feature of the second phase of the attack. At this point increased pressure on certain parts of the brain might produce feelings of nausea.

The ALCAT Test measures the change in the size and number of white blood cells and also identifies when foods or chemicals cause platelet clumping. (This serotonin-induced constriction of the vasculature may explain how fenfluramine [of "phen-fen" fame] and its related compound, dexfenfluramine [trade name Redux] lead to an increased risk for primary pulmonary hypertension [PPH] and associated heart valve damage.)

Flawed Theories

Two popular theories regarding how severe headaches and migraines come about relate to specific food "triggers" and hormonal changes. Yet eliminating foods such as chocolate, aged cheese, and red wine and taking hormone-managing drugs such as nonsteroidal, anti-inflammatory agents have helped few sufferers. The "amines" in certain foods are thought to affect the diameter of the blood vessels, and thereby produce headaches. (Amines are byproducts of chemical reactions involving amino acids in the body, but also exist naturally in certain foods. The most common reference is to foods high in tyramine. Tyramine is neutralized in the bodies of most people by monamine oxidase.)

But research has shown that "there must be other factors that can make the platelets clump together, because it is only a minority of patients whose migraines are triggered by these foods," says Dr. Brostoff. He continues by describing the process:

> The foods identified by an elimination diet seem to be acting in a different way from the accepted food "triggers." When these foods are eliminated from the diet, the migraines usually clear up completely, whereas excluding trigger foods only makes the migraines less frequent. Following an elimination diet, and the avoidance of culprit foods, patients often find that they can once more tolerate their triggers—both food and nonfood. It looks as if the milk, wheat, or whatever was creating some serious underlying problem that made the body vulnerable to any external change.
>
> Thus bright lights, stress, the flickering of a television screen, or the pharmacologically active substances in chocolate could upset the delicate balance and tip the whole system into a migraine attack. Once the underlying food intolerance has been sorted out, the system is far more stable

and can better cope with external circumstances. . . . One of the main preventive measures is to minimize the "load" by excluding the worst offenders or minimizing the lesser offenders. There is a threshold beyond which a migraine attack is triggered; to lower the load so that the threshold is never reached enables the individual to maintain health rather than to have to treat an illness.

Eliminating our system's reactive foods is the fastest, most effective way to reduce the "load" on our system.

Hormonal changes have also been implicated as a cause of migraines due to the fact that migraines affect women more than men, and they often begin occurring at the onset of menstruation. However, if female endocrine changes are to blame, the current treatment of choice—drugs—is a poor solution for most people. According to an article in the January/February 1996 issue of *Health* magazine, written by Dr. Fred Sheftell, director and co-founder of the New England Center for Headache, the migraine pharmaceuticals don't work for everyone, and can have dangerous side effects. Interestingly, the drugs mimic the neurotransmitter serotonin by constricting blood vessels. However, the drugs show no discretion in which blood vessels they constrict; along with brain blood vessels, they constrict blood vessels leading to the heart, legs, and arms—which can lead to potentially severe health problems.

"If you're born with this disorder, it's like having a stick of dynamite with a fuse in your head, and certain activators—stress, foods, hormonal fluctuations—light it," Dr. Sheftell says. The article further reported that migraine sufferers are waiting for the "breakthrough drug" or the "perfect fix" that will block migraines by reducing the inflammation in their head without affecting arteries or veins in other parts of the body. They just don't know yet that thousands of migraine sufferers have *already* discovered the perfect fix—eliminating intolerant foods. What could be safer or more natural than that?

Further, patients are rarely aware of the environmental source of their illness. You may see no relation between eating and your headaches, because the effects can be delayed (from one hour to seven days). Or you may know that your headache is somehow related to food intake, but that intake is so complex and varied that uncovering the actual source may seem impossible. Or you may know that a particular food *relieves* your headache pain, not realizing that the "relief" meal is nothing but your maintenance dose.

Serotonin is a chemical substance primarily present in the platelets. This neurotransmitter, which is also naturally produced in the brain, has the job of sending messages between nerve cells, thereby controlling how we feel. Serotonin may have different effects when it is produced in the brain to serve as a neurotransmitter as opposed to being released into the bloodstream as a result of an inflammatory reaction and platelet clumping. Vasodilatation may be viewed as the body's tendency to return to normal following the vasoconstriction associated with a food reaction and platelet clumping.

As Dr. Solomon puts it: "With any condition, unless you remove all the foods that trigger a person's migraines, you're not going to get to the problem."

CHAPTER 14

Food Intolerance: How to Live With It

Once you know or suspect food intolerance, the treatment is avoiding offending food. In our fast-food, multiethnic food-oriented society, this can be quite a challenge. Treatment of food intolerance requires commitment and focus. For the most part, you will need to prepare foods at home to be sure reactive foods are carefully excluded. This can be an imposition if you eat most meals out. That doesn't change the fact that you must eliminate your offending foods before your symptoms will subside.

Eat Safely

The most practical approach to eliminating reactive foods is to assimilate a list of "safe" foods. Such a list is provided along with ALCAT Test results. Your ALCAT list of foods is divided into four parts, each containing representative foods from each major food family to be eaten on four consecutive days. This helps you plan meals in which no food is repeated more frequently than every four days, yet ensures that you'll get the needed vitamins and minerals to maintain good nutrient health. By using the "safe" foods in this way, you minimize intolerance to new foods and achieve variety and diversity by exploring new food choices rather than coveting your old favorites.

While following your elimination diet, you'll find it best to stick to simple basic meals and avoid complicated recipes and dishes, which concentrate too many food choices in a single meal and often severely limit later meal choices. After about two weeks, you might anticipate improvement of any symptoms associated with food intolerance. Any symptoms associated with reactive foods will continue to subside if you continue to avoid foods to which you are sensitive.

Become a Detective

If some symptoms linger, you may need to further eliminate suspicious foods, probably those that are a regular part of your diet. You might, for example, eliminate wheat, corn, milk, peanuts, tomatoes, and soy if you haven't already eliminated them. Although others may well be the real culprits, the ones mentioned are so insidious in American processed foods that they easily slip into elimination diets. Strategically eliminating these foods in conjunction with your known reactive foods may lead to relief of your symptoms. At this point, you might contact a professional acquainted with strict elimination diets to help you seek out the culprit food.

A curious and as yet unexplained phenomenon of food sensitivity is that you may need to eliminate all your reactive foods before your symptoms will subside because they may represent reactions to food combinations rather than to individual foods. For that reason, eliminating individual reactive foods one at a time and using relief of symptoms as your endpoint is not a reliable method.

Should you test positive to a large number of foods, rather than assume the imposing task of eliminating this mass of favorite foods in one swift stroke, choosing five or six foods to eliminate the first week is less painful. Then you can add more foods to your elimination list for the second week and so on until you have included all your reactive foods. This method allows you to adapt to your new diet without the shock of losing all your standby foods at once. Nonetheless, you must eliminate all your reactive foods at the same time to expect the best results.

Identify Your Reactive Foods

You'll find the ALCAT Test results in an informative guide to your reactive foods. You will find a complete list of all the foods tested in the front of the guide. Each food will be accompanied by a rating of either "negative," "1+", "2+," or "MPOS."

The "negative" foods are those to which you demonstrate no allergic reaction. These represent your "safe" foods and should be the foundation of your diet plan as you eliminate your reactive foods.

The "1+" foods are those to which you exhibited a reaction, but of an equivocal nature. That is to say, only a small percentage of the white blood cells and/or platelets showed signs of response. These foods may represent potential intolerance, but for the most part should be consumed cautiously. Eating these foods no more often than once a week will allow you to determine whether or not they contribute to your symptoms. If you had very few foods in the "2+" or "MPOS" range, you should eliminate those in the "1+" range. Reactive foods may fall into the "1+" range erroneously if you were taking certain anti-inflammatory medications, antihistamines, or steroids when the test was administered.

If you are not losing weight by exercising regularly and are hungry after exercising, consider testing for food sensitivities.

Foods in the "2+" range are those to which you are likely to be intolerant. Curiously, you may find some foods in this category that you rarely or never eat. Because this may represent genetically determined intolerance, you are wise to continue to avoid these foods. Foods in the "2+" range represent foods to which your cells exhibited significant signs of reaction. You should eliminate these foods from your diet meticulously for a period of at least three months, after which you may reintroduce them into your diet to evaluate its intolerance. Food intolerance is different from allergic reactions in that the body may cease to react to the food after a period of elimination. When reintroducing foods, add only one food at a time. Eat normal quantities of this food on a single day, then wait three days before you reintroduce any others. If no characteristic symptoms develop, you may incorporate the food into your four-day rotation diet plan.

Foods in the "MPOS" range represent those foods that elicited the maximum positive reaction from your body's cells. These foods, like those in the "2+" range, should be strictly eliminated for a period of at least three months before you attempt to reintroduce them. Keep in mind that the degree of reactivity does not accurately establish the cause of symptoms. Symptoms may result from any of your reactive foods. The degrees of reaction only represent the intensity with which your blood cells reacted to a particular food in the test.

In many cases, individual reactive foods may cause symptoms only when they are eaten along with other reactive foods; the combination of these foods may cause you problems. Strictly avoiding all your reactive foods is the most practical way to eliminate food allergy symptoms.

Avoid Your Intolerant Foods

Following the report of your degree of reactivity to various foods is a concise listing of your reactive foods and their close relatives. This is a useful list to copy and keep in the car, purse or briefcase, and kitchen. Having this list available at strategic times when you are shopping or preparing food will lessen the likelihood of inadvertently eating foods you should eliminate.

You will notice that class 1+ reactive foods do not appear on this list unless you had very few 2+ or MPOS foods. You should consider class 1+ reactive foods "equivocal" unless they are the predominant reactive category. If class 1+ foods appear here, you should eliminate them completely because they may represent the maximum reaction the body is able to muster under certain conditions. Also, keep in mind that using anti-inflammatory medication, steroids, and antihistamines may alter the body's reaction to an allergen.

Stick to Your Eating List

This list of "safe" foods that should make up the foundation of your diet plan is your gold mine. Foods to which you tested negative are unlikely to be reactive for you. Take some time to carefully review this list. Most represent staples you are familiar with or reasonable substitutes you may never have tried because the local grocery didn't find them profitable. It is important to begin to realize how much we are at the mercy of the retailer's bottom line when we shop for food.

Don't be put off by the sometimes unusual names. Most foods on this list can be found at progressive grocers or at health-food stores. You will soon appreciate this if you are intolerant of common foods such as corn, wheat, milk, eggs, or soy. Our packaged food industry makes prolific use of common foods—in fact, about 75 percent of the foods in a package at a grocery contain corn or corn products. No wonder corn shows up on the list of ten foods to which people are most likely to be intolerant. Use this information to realize how important it is to vary your foods from day to day.

Follow a Four-Day Rotation Diet

This section conveniently separates all your "safe" foods into four consecutive days to ensure you will not eat any one food more than once in the four-day cycle. It is a useful way to juggle the large list of foods you may eat. There is nothing sacred about the particular arrangement of these foods, and you may switch foods to different days if you wish. The important thing to remember is that once you switch a food, you should eat it no more often than every fourth day to minimize the prospect of developing new food intolerance while on your elimination diet.

General Information

What follows in the manual is a computer-generated information section to assist you in planning your meals. Understand that this section does not take into account your individual food intolerance. You should read this section only to reinforce your dietary planning—not to justify eating a food to which you are reactive.

Your Reactive Food Information

I consider this section the most informative in the manual. Here you will learn more about your reactive foods and how to avoid them, than you will ever need to know. Full of insights to avoid ruining your elimination diet plan, this section bears careful attention.

Treating Candida Albicans

This particular reactive test is worth discussing separately. If you tested positive to *candida,* you will have noticed that the list of foods you are allowed is exceptionally small. This is because all sugars, starches, and yeast-containing foods have been eliminated.

Candida survives in your intestine by living on simple carbohydrates. Eliminating this food supply is necessary to kill the yeast. Testing positive to candida means that your immune system detected the organism in your bloodstream at some time. Candida can spread via the bloodstream to other organs and become a serious life-threatening problem in cases of a severely compromised immune system (such as during chemotherapy or in persons with cancer). The fact that candida was detected in your bloodstream at all justifies aggressive dietary treatment. Many physicians prefer aggressive drug treatment of candida at the time of dietary restriction, so you may want to consult with your physician regarding this. An excellent resource for those testing positive to candida is *The Yeast Connection* by William Crook, M.D.

Taking the Challenge Test

The challenge test is a mechanism for testing previously eliminated foods to evaluate their reactivity (or tendency to cause symptoms). This is accomplished by meticulously eliminating a food for a period of greater than two weeks, by which time your body will react differently if you are truly reactive to the food. When you reintroduce the food after two weeks of elimination, the typical reaction may be of a hyper-reactive nature—more immediate and more intense than previously noticed. For this reason it is best to challenge only test foods that were equivocal in their allerginicity (1+). Paying careful attention to your symptoms for the next three days should establish the safety index of the food. If a food does not elicit reactions when challenge tested, you may include it in your four-day elimination diet plan. However, if challenge testing a food results in return of your symptoms, strictly eliminate the food from the diet for a period of three to six months before you repeat challenge testing. If a food persists in precipitating symptoms after three months, you should eliminate it for one year before retesting.

The good news is that much food intolerance resolves after three months of strict elimination. The exact mechanism for this is not known. Remember that people with food intolerance tend toward food intolerance in the future. The practice of rotating foods on a four-day schedule is useful in decreasing the likelihood of your food intolerances reoccurring.

The above descriptions of food elimination and challenge testing are particularly applicable if you present the overt physical symptoms often associated with food intolerance. If your primary symptom of food intolerance is overweight, you must take a different approach.

In case of food intolerance as a cause of overweight, the culprit foods should be eliminated for three months. Then they should be reintroduced only on a four-day rotating basis. Challenge testing is not beneficial if the only physical evidence of intolerance is overweight. It is relatively easy to notice the sudden onset of sinus congestion, headache, or fatigue, but quite another to evaluate a subtle change in weight when you are challenge-testing a food.

Talk will not conquer obesity as a public health menace. Drugs have not decreased deaths from obesity. It is time for the individual to guide his or her health care and destiny relating to weight. Take a proactive position regarding your health by learning how to identify and eliminate your reactive foods. Congratulations on your major commitment to protect your health through the elimination of your reactive foods.

"Let Thy Food Be Thy Medicine"

No single aspect of American life influences our health more than does the food we eat. As we finally set out to eliminate overweight and its incredible burden on society, our focus must be on the food we eat and its relationship to the diseases that kill us prematurely. Our food makes many of us fat because we react inappropriately to it.

According to the March 9, 1998, *PRNewswire,* James M. Rippe, M.D., of the Center for Clinical and Lifestyle Research and Tufts University School of Medicine, urges physicians to treat obesity as an independent health problem rather than simply treating its common consequences—such as coronary heart disease, hypertension,

Type 2 diabetes, and elevated blood lipids. Dr. Rippe emphasized that while data clearly support the positive effects of weight loss on reducing health risk, physicians have not taken an active role in treating obesity. He also states: "Traditionally, physicians have failed to treat obesity in their patients. . . . Identifying patients early and starting long-term obesity treatment including diet, exercise and new pharmacotherapies when appropriate can save lives. We must attack obesity to attack the root of the problem."

As this book establishes, unrecognized and untreated food intolerance is a cause of overweight, as well as a cause of migraine headaches, sinus congestion, attention-deficit disorder, arthritis, fatigue, irritable bowel syndrome, colitis, gastritis, skin rashes, and depression. Yet as we search for an explanation of overweight, it will almost certainly be outside the traditional concepts of conventional medical philosophy. Years of research and study have failed to explain why people lose and regain unwanted weight except to note people gain weight when they eat too much.

But we can now keep the wild animal inside of us at bay. Without spending weeks trying and trading foods to determine which may be causing our problems, we can put information in front of us by taking the ALCAT Test. By avoiding the reactive foods the test identifies, we re-open doors long since shut in our face. Again in control, we can watch our weight melt away as our cravings disappear and food no longer holds our mind hostage. Clean out the cupboards, review basic nutrition, and cull bad habits; it's a whole new lifestyle. So redeeming is the freedom from the limitations of food intolerance that the words from the old spiritual quoted by Reverend Martin Luther King come to mind: "Free at last, free at last, thank God Almighty, free at last."

Food elimination as a cure for disease, often referred to as "alternative medicine," now takes the spotlight by default. Nothing else has worked. Again we appreciate the value of the earliest medical advice given 2,500 years ago by Hippocrates, the father of medicine: "Let thy food be thy medicine and thy medicine be thy food." The science and art of eliminating or prescribing food for the relief of illness has always been medicinal. Conventional intervention might better be considered "alternative medicine." Identifying and eliminating intolerant foods is the new "medicine" to conquer obesity.

Frequently Asked Questions
about Food Sensitivities

Food intolerance represents a new and radical reform in health care that conflicts with many conventional concepts of food and eating. These conventional approaches have perpetuated overweight and confused the general population. Following are answers to some of the commonly asked questions regarding the cause and treatment of overweight.

Q **Doctor, I exercise regularly and try to eat healthy, but I can't seem to lose weight. Could food sensitivities be part of my problem?**

A Yes, food intolerance may well be a part of your problem in losing weight. Normally when we exercise we tap into our fat stores for energy. Aerobic exercise is the best form of exercise to consume fat because fat must be oxidized to utilize it as energy. Therefore exercise classified as aerobic (that is, "with air") would be the best choice of exercise if one's goal were to decrease body fat stores. In the case of food-intolerant individuals, the chemical reaction of the allergic food seems to prevent the efficient use of fat for energy.

The exact mechanism of this has yet to be determined, but if you tend to become increasingly hungry after exercise, your body is telling you that your exercise was financed with your emergency energy stores of glycogen, emergency energy stores found in your liver and muscle. Once you have tapped these emergency stores, your body will insist that you replenish this energy as soon as possible to be ready for the next emergency. Needless to say, this is not the ideal energy source for someone trying to lose fat weight by exercising. In fact, a number of patients gained fat as well as muscle weight when they began exercise programs. This was a result of their increased hunger after exercise, which they tended to satisfy with carbohydrate and fat snacks. The end result was that the fat was stored and became part of the problem they were trying to eliminate.

Fortunately, once they eliminated foods to which they were intolerant, they began to notice more appropriate changes in their body composition (lean tissue to fat ratio) in response to regular aerobic exercise. As an added bonus, they were not hungry after exercise because they did not have to replenish their emergency energy stores. Exercise should alleviate hunger, not make it worse. If you are not losing fat weight by exercising regularly and are hungry after exercising, consider testing for food sensitivities.

Q **Using medication I can consistently lose weight for a couple of months but as soon as I stop the medication I start gaining it back. Should I just stay on the medicine permanently?**

A If anyone requires medication permanently, their doctor has apparently exhausted all other means to diagnose and treat their condition. As far as I know, no one who is overweight suffers from low blood levels of appetite suppressants any more than headache is caused by aspirin deficiency. So, taking them on a permanent basis is probably not the best solution to the problem. Before you give up, be sure that you and your doctor are delving into all the possible causes of your overweight. These may include candidiasis, thyroid disorders, pituitary disorders, genetically inherited disorders, poor eating habits, nutritional deficiencies, emotional eating, stress eating, and obviously food intolerance. (The list is actually longer but you get the idea.) The odds are that with nutritional guidance and real lifestyle changes, you can probably deal with the problem of overweight without the crutch of appetite suppressants. Find a doctor who is interested in eliminating all the likely underlying causes of your overweight.

Q **I can't seem to lose weight after my doctor stopped giving me Pondomin and recently found a source of Pondomin from Mexico. Would it be okay for me to take it from time to time?**

A No. There is no good reason to risk your health taking a drug that has been taken off the market in America. Our health-care system may have many faults, but ignoring evidence that a drug may be dangerous to use would be foolish and irresponsible.

Find a doctor who will help you discover the underlying cause of your overweight and treat it appropriately. The quick fix is always a bad idea. The lifestyle we live in America is so fast paced that we often don't spend time taking care of ourselves. The price we pay is a lifetime of frustration with frequent quick trips to the doctor. Until we become responsible for our actions and treat our bodies with respect, medicine is not going to be the answer. Real treatment of any disease involves the partnership of your doctor's knowledge and your commitment to become healthy.

Q **Doctor, I have severe adult acne, terrible migraine headaches, and am about 75 pounds overweight. No one has been able to help me with these problems. How come our medical system that can transplant hearts can't do more for my problems?**

A To dissect the politics and economics of medicine in this country is beyond the scope of this response. Suffice it to say that your doctors haven't yet found the underlying cause of your problems. Although all of your conditions may be related to food sensitivities, there certainly are a variety of other possible etiologies. Nonetheless, if you haven't been tested for food sensitivities, it would be worthwhile to do so. Many people find that eliminating reactive foods gives them long overdue relief from chronic conditions thought to be incurable.

Q **Doctor, how can you be so sure that food sensitivities are the cause of overweight?**

A I can't be sure that food sensitivities are the cause of everyone's overweight. Overweight has become a national stigma and its "cause" has evaded definition to date. I do know that weight loss evaded many of my patients until they eliminated foods identified by sensitivity testing. We all know that eating too much food will lead to overweight. What we may be overlooking is that in some cases "too much" may be only a bite of the wrong food. Food intolerance as a cause of overweight makes remarkable good sense—as the "cause of the cause" of overweight. That is, food intolerance results in overeating of foods which, although they increase serotonin levels, also increase fat deposits. That answer was a bit more complicated than I like, but I'm sure you get the idea.

Q **Doctor, do you think I can lose weight if I find out what foods I am sensitive to?**

A I am pretty sure you will *not* lose weight if you *only* find out to which foods you are sensitive. To benefit from knowledge of food intolerance, you must eliminate the culprit foods, and this means *ELIMINATE* in most cases. If you are unable to completely eliminate the culprit foods for the necessary period of time, allowing your body to "forget" the sensitivity, you may well suffer relapses. This can be avoided by seeking the help of a professional who can advise you as to "challenge testing" (introducing foods one at a time to see whether you still react adversely to a food) as well as healthy nutritional balance to prevent the likelihood of acquiring new food intolerance.

Q **Doctor, I know my reactive foods, but my weight loss seems slow, only a pound or two each week. Is there anything I can do to speed this up?**

A First of all, my calculations show that at a pound or two each week, you would lose between 50 and 100 pounds a year, which is plenty of weight to lose in a year. The need for immediate gratification is a fault we are all guilty of from time to time. Practical healthy physiologic limits to weight loss permit all the involved body systems to synchronize their functions as the burden of overweight is removed.

Rather than fixating on weight loss per se, you would do well to sit down with a health professional you respect and identify your eating triggers—emotional eating, stress eating, pleasure eating, for example. Make a plan for healthy lifestyle changes that will maintain your successful weight loss. Implementing these changes gradually as you lose weight will give you the confidence needed to keep the weight off. It is important to discover and resolve all the precipitating forces involved in overeating to prevent relapse.

Q **Doctor, I am having trouble finding foods that taste good to me on my elimination diet; I am attracted to my familiar foods. Is it okay for me to mix some of my reactive foods with my "safe" foods to give them some taste?**

A Nice try, but sorry, you must eliminate your reactive foods to prevent the allergic reaction in your body. Sneaking or "accidentally on purpose" eating your reactive foods will result in having to start over the necessary elimination period. Curiously, you may find that you experience a hyperacute reaction to these foods if you eat them before your body has completely given them the seal of approval. This means you may experience an intense, rapid reaction after eating the food that had been incompletely eliminated. From my experience, such a reaction is great incentive to stick to your elimination diet.

If you eliminate saturated fats and all sweets during your elimination time frame, you will find that natural foods taste different and better than you remembered. It seems that fats and sugar are so stimulating to the taste buds that nothing else can quite compare. This leads us to search for more fats and sugar to equal the taste "intoxication" mode of eating. How often have you heard someone rave so about a fatty, sugary treat that you would think it was as healthy as mother's milk? They are eating for taste to the exclusion of nutrition.

Q If I can never eat these foods again, what will I do if I develop intolerance to the foods I am allowed?

A Good question. First of all, remember that for some reason not completely understood, the immune system often "forgets" a delayed food allergy if it doesn't come in contact with the food for a period of time. This may represent an eccentricity of the immune system that allowed early man to feast on foods in season. When not available, man essentially eliminated them from his diet and never suffered the long-term effects of food intolerance. In modern times, we must work at eliminating foods from the diet because they are available year-round. It is generally recognized that after a period of three to six months, reactive foods may be reintroduced into the diet. To decide whether a food remains reactive, it is reintroduced in normal amounts and observed for renewal of symptoms for a period of three days. It is important to "challenge" test only one food at a time. An alternative would be to repeat the ALCAT Test every three to six months.

Secondly, it is important to avoid the development of new food intolerance while on your elimination diet. This is accomplished by eating slowly, varying your foods through rotation diet planning, enhancing immune system nutrition through diet and supplements, and doing something to alleviate the stress in your life.

Q **I have lost weight using a commercial weight-loss program, but regained the weight soon after leaving the program. How would food intolerance explain this?**

A Most commercial weight-loss programs focus on calorie reduction and exercise to effect weight loss. Until the underlying causes of overweight are identified and treated, the condition is likely to recur. Food intolerance may play a role in these programs in that the diets and supplements prescribed are a "one-size-fits-all" program. That is, their profit is to be made from sales of food and food supplements and exchanges designed to lower caloric intake overall. This is without regard for food intolerance. If an individual is intolerant of a food or a food component of the supplement, weight loss and maintenance is going to be unlikely. Likewise if the individual eliminates his reactive food for only a short period of time, the allergic reaction will likely resume as he or she resumes their "regular" diet.

Any weight-loss program can be enhanced through the use of the ALCAT Test to identify reactive foods. You should eliminate these foods in addition to the other modalities to effectively lose and keep weight off.

Q **Why do I crave some of the foods I am sensitive to?**

A This curious aspect of food intolerance is not yet well understood, though some suggest it may represent withdrawal. When the chemical reactions precipitated by the allergic response are pleasurable, the absence of this allergic response results in unpleasant feelings, which can only be remedied by eating the food and creating the allergic reaction again.

Another interesting theory compares food sensitivities to serum sickness. The body produces excessive antibodies to a food such that the individual is actually sick from their own antibodies. Only when the food antigen is reintroduced and binds with the antibodies does the condition improve. Unfortunately the food stimulates more antibodies and the cycle repeats.

More research is needed to define this aspect of food sensitivities. Until the answers are in, your best efforts should be directed toward eliminating your reactive foods.

Q **My two brothers and my mother are allergic to wheat. Am I likely to be allergic to wheat also?**

A Maybe. Evidence suggests that some food intolerance may be genetically programmed. Although each individual is different, certain tendencies are genetically predetermined. For example, if one's ancestors never developed the enzyme systems to metabolize milk byproducts, the body may protect itself from toxic overload through allergic response to discourage drinking of milk in all its descendants. Interesting observations in Denmark have revealed similar sensitivities in identical twins. Although this is interesting, thorough testing is still necessary to determine one's food sensitivities. Further study is necessary to establish any useful predictive value to one family member's food intolerance.

Q **How I can be sensitive to a food I have never eaten?**

A This question comes up frequently as we review test results with patients. The answer again lies in genetic predisposition. People may be genetically programmed to be intolerant of a food. This may occur without their ever having been exposed to the food. The good news is that if one has never been exposed to the food, it is obviously not a favorite food and therefore not a problem to eliminate. Genetically modulated food intolerances are, however, of a more permanent nature than immune system modulated intolerances. If you find you are intolerant of a food you don't ever remember eating, you will probably always have a reaction to that food. So, it would be best to continue not eating it. Be aware, however, that the food in question may be present in some prepared foods without your realizing it.

Q My seasonal pollen allergies have improved tremendously since I have eliminated my reactive foods. Can food allergies make pollen allergies worse?

A Many patients realize an improvement in symptoms of airborne allergies after eliminating reactive foods. In some cases the mechanism may be one of cross-reactivity. We know, for example, that sensitivity to apples is predictive of sensitivity to Birch pollen, and sensitivity to cantaloupe is often coupled with sensitivity to ragweed. Once the food sensitivity is resolved, the airborne allergy may also improve or disappear.

Another interesting aspect of food intolerance is the relationship of co-factors. You may not typically react to a food but may react to the same food if you eat it following exercise. Or you may only react to a food seasonally when certain pollen co-factors are present. Often another food is the inciting co-factor, without which there is no apparent reaction. This aspect of food intolerance is a "gray area" but symptomatically responds well to removal of either of the co-factor components.

Q My elimination diet leaves me very little food that I care to eat. Would I be able to use the protein drinks at the health-food stores as meal substitutes until I can re-introduce some of my foods?

A I would encourage you to explore the many foods listed as the foods you may eat. Although these may seem strange to you, I believe you will find them not unlike their common cousins, to which you are more accustomed. Expanding your food choices is a benefit in terms of nutrition.

Commercially prepared protein meal substitutes are generally not a good idea on your elimination diet. These commercial concoctions are more often than not made from a wide variety of substances known to be allergenic. The protein in these meal replacements is usually derived from egg, soy, and milk protein, all of which are high on the list of common reactive substances. To make matters worse, many of these formulas contain large amounts of hidden sugars and chemicals to improve the taste.

If a packaged meal substitute were needed for traveling or just to avoid the inconvenience of preparing food during the day, the ATML Corp. has available a hypoallergenic protein formula. This proprietary formula is a rich and healthy protein base, chemical-free and vitamin-enriched, which is more appropriate for the food-intolerant individual. Taste-wise it is better than most protein meal substitutes and is appropriate for anyone not intolerant of rice.

Fast track to staying well.   If you get sick, assume it was something you ate that you shouldn't have or something you didn't eat that you should have; and don't do it again.

BIBLIOGRAPHY OF SELECTED ALCAT TEST STUDIES

The studies below are a sampling of international ALCAT Test studies and results that confirm the effectiveness of the Test.

Cabo-Soler, J. R. Comments on diets in esthetic medicine. Presented at the 14th Mediterranean Day of Esthetical Medicine and Dermatological Surgery, Venice, Italy, Sept. 22–23, 1995.

This Spanish study was designed to determine whether people who could not lose weight on a low calorie diet could resume their weight loss using the results from the ALCAT Test.

Using a group of 30 patients who had difficulty losing weight when they adhered to a reduced calorie diet, this study confirmed a greater weight loss in almost all the patients when they were placed on a diet planned according to the ALCAT Test results. Also, the weight loss was mostly fat, with minor muscle loss. In some cases, muscle mass was increased.

Other interesting observations included (1) improved skin smoothness, (2) a loss of fat from the thigh area, making it useful in planning a diet to control cellulitis, (3) a better sense of well being and improved physical performance, and (4) improvement in abdominal bloating and digestive problems.

These findings are significant because many overweight patients find it difficult to lose weight by cutting calories alone. This study suggests that delayed food allergies may interfere with weight loss regardless of calorie restriction. Also, the beneficial effects of skin smoothness, loss of fat from the thigh area, improved sense of well being, and improvement of gastrointestinal conditions were bonuses to those following the ALCAT diet plan

Fell, P., J. Brostoff, and M. Pasula. "High Correlation of the ALCAT Test Results with Double-Blind Challenge in Food Sensitivity." Paper presented at the 45th annual Congress of the American College of Allergy and Immunology, Nov. 12–16, 1988. Published in *Annals of Allergy.*

This double-blind American study was designed to determine the reliability of ALCAT Test results. Double-blind studies mean that neither researchers nor participants know who is receiving treatment and who is not. This method assures an impartial assessment of the participants.

This study was designed to test the accuracy of the ALCAT Test versus a traditional double-blind challenge with the same foods. (For the 58 ALCAT positive foods selected from the 19 subjects, 46 were positive on double-blind challenge [79.3 percent] and 12 were negative. Of the 56 ALCAT negative foods, 49 were also negative by double blind challenge [87.5 percent] and 7 were positive.) Overall correlation between the ALCAT Test and the double-blind challenge was 83.4 percent, suggesting the ALCAT Test was quite reliable in identifying unsafe foods in these sensitive subjects.

Høj, L. "Diagnostic Value of the ALCAT Test in Intolerance to Food Additives Compared with Double-Blind Placebo-Controlled Oral Challenges." Paper presented at the 52nd annual meeting of the American Academy of Allergy, Asthma, and Immunology, March 15–20, 1996. Published in *Journal of Allergy and Clinical Immunology*, Vol. 97, no.1, part 3, Jan. 1996.

This Danish study was designed to determine whether the ALCAT Test could consistently detect intolerance to food additives. Using 26 randomly chosen patients with known food additive intolerances, 76 food addictive challenges were done using the double-blind technique. The ALCAT Test predicted negative and positive reactions with 95 percent accuracy.

———. "Food Intolerance in Patients with Angioedema and Chronic Urticaria: An Investigation by Rast and ALCAT Test." Paper presented at the XVI European Congress of Allergology and Clinical Immunology, Madrid, Spain, June 25–30, 1995. Published in *European Journal of Allergy and Clinical Immunology*, Supplement No. 26, Vol. 50, 1995.

This test confirmed the effectiveness of ALCAT testing over Rast testing in determining the cause of angioedema (swelling) and urticaria (hives). This study also confirmed the importance of food sensitivities as a cause of allergic reactions and hives.

This Danish study used 52 patients to test the hypothesis of food intolerance being associated with chronic urticaria (itching) and angioedema (swelling). When patients' individual diets consisted of foods to which (according to the ALCAT Test) they showed no sensitivity, there was complete remission of both angioedema and urticaria in 45 patients, remission of angioedema but not urticaria in five, and failure in one.

Kaats, G., D. Pullen, and L. Parker. "The Short-Term Efficacy of the ALCAT Test to Facilitate Changes in Body Composition and Self-Reported Disease Symptoms: A Randomized Study." *The Bariatrician*, Spring 1996.

This Texas study evaluated the benefits of supplying dieters with information about their food sensitivities.

Subjects had body composition measurements taken and were given a disease symptom questionnaire. They were then separated into two groups, with one group being given a diet plan based on their ALCAT results. The other group (the control group) was asked to pursue a weight-loss plan of their own choosing.

Results showed the ALCAT group lost significantly more pounds, body fat percentage, and body fat weight than the control group. The ALCAT group also reported improvements in all 20 symptoms listed in the disease symptom questionnaire.

Pasula, M., and S. Puccio. "Multiple Pathogenic Mechanisms in Food Sensitivity Reactions In-Vitro." Presented at the 4th International Symposium on Immunological and Clinical Problems of Food Allergy, Milan, Italy. Nov 5–9, 1989. Published in the proceedings.

This study evaluated the multiple pathogenic pathways involved in food allergy reactions. Whole blood from nine food-sensitive asthmatic patients was incubated with each extract, and immunoglobulin levels were measured. Significant changes in one or more immunoglobulin and complement component occurred in every patient to one or more foods. The ALCAT Test was shown to be effective in identifying these food sensitivities.

Sandberg, D., and M. Pasula. "A Comparison of the ALCAT Test for Food Reactions Amongst Two Population Subgroups." Presented at the 45th Annual Congress of the American College of Allergy and Immunology, Los Angeles, Calif. Nov. 12–16, 1988. Published in *Annals of Allergy*.

This study was designed to test whether the ALCAT Test can discriminate between a healthy group and a group with food allergies. The study used a control group of 25 healthy young athletes with no history of food sensitivities and an age-matched group of 25 young people with suspected food sensitivities. Of the 225 reactions observed for each group, the healthy group had a total of 5 positive reactions compared to 45 reactions for the patient group.

Solomon, B. "The ALCAT Test: A Guide and Barometer in the Therapy of Environmental and Food Sensitivities." *Environmental Medicine*, Vol. 9, No. 2, 1992.

This study reviewed 172 individuals one to two years after they began diets based on the results of their ALCAT Tests. An independent reviewer asked patients to evaluate the effect of food elimination and/or allergy shots on their symptoms on a scale of 1 to 10.

Results confirmed the value of the ALCAT Test and the elimination diet in alleviating symptoms such as migraine, sinus congestion, irritable bowel, gastrointestinal reflux, arthritis, asthma, fatigue, obesity, and eczema.

Steinman, H., M.D., Department of Clinical Science and Immunology, Medical School, University of Cape Town, South Africa. Unpublished study, 1997.

In this South African study, 12 patients were tested using the ALCAT Test for each of 50 foods. Each test was done in duplicate or triplicate samples, resulting in 94.4 percent reproducibility of the data. In addition to the high reproducibility of the scores, two patients suffering from gastrointestinal symptoms had dramatic improvement of their symptoms following an elimination diet constructed with the aid of the ALCAT Test.

INDEX

Absorptive malnutrition, 122
Acid reflux, 151, 208
Acne, 21, 244–246
  adult acne, 301–302
Adaptive immune system, 91–92
Addiction to foods, 197–199
Adenosine deaminase, 87
Adipose tissue, 200
Adkins high protein diet, 144
Adrenaline, 249
Aerobic exercise, 208
  benefits of, 299
  cellulite prevention and, 252
African Americans, lactase deficiency in, 100
AIDS/HIV, 87
Airborne allergies, 92–96
  elimination of reactive foods and, 307
Air pollution, 75
ALCAT test, 8, 20–22, 40, 60, 97, 160–161, 179–181
  case study, 168–169
  deciding on, 173–175
  evolution of, 22–24
  experiences of doctors, 198–199
  immune system and, 89–90
  infections and, 11–12
  infertility issues, 10–11

international studies and
  results, 309–313
leukocytes in, 105–106
lists of food types, 290–292
normals in, 186, 210
safe foods, identifying, 134
serotonin and, 58–60
track record of, 209–210
Alcohol use, 22
  blood types and alcoholism, 98
  candida and, 124
  cellulite prevention and, 251–252
  gastrointestinal tract and, 225
  overeating and, 123
Allergen-specific antibodies, 95
Allergic airway disease, 226
Allergic reaction, 151–152, 154
Allergies. *See also* Airborne allergies; Hay fever
  classic allergic reaction, 92
  etymology of term, 91
  true allergy, 91
All-you-can-eat specials, 130
Alpha2 receptors, 249–250
An Alternative Approach to Allergies (Randolph), 257, 273–274
Alternative medicine, 80
American Dietetic Association, 72

American Medical Testing Laboratories, 24
Amines, 285
Amino acids
obesity and, 56–57
serotonin and, 116
AMTL Company, 220
Anaphylactic shock, 6, 86
Anger, overeating and, 183
Angioedema, 242, 244
percent improvement in, 245
Angiograms, 74
Antibiotics, 81
candidiasis and, 124, 125
gastrointestinal tract and, 225
Antibodies, 94
Antidepressants, 146
Antigen-presenting cells, 93
Antihistamines, 292
Anti-inflammatory medications
allergens, reactions to, 292
for asthma, 230
non-steroidal anti-
inflammatories (NSAIDs),
225
Anxiety, 21
Appetite suppressants, 48, 146
hunger and, 148
nutrition and, 148–149
track record of, 206–207
Arachidonic acid, 201
Arthritis, 6, 8–9, 21, 152, 297
yo-yo dieting and, 42
Asian Americans, lactase deficiency in, 100
Aspartame, 140
Aspirin, 83
avoidance of, 225
Asthma, 21, 208, 231–232
case history, 227–228
exercise and, 22
food allergies and, 235
increase in rates of, 229–230
obesity and, 35
research on, 234–235
symptoms of, 229–230

Astragalus, 218
Atherosclerosis, 13–14
immune system and, 90
ATML Corp., 308
Atopy, 95
Attention deficit disorder (ADD),
5, 18, 297
case study, 169–170
foods causing, 170–171
Attention deficit hyperactivity dis-
order (ADHD), 18, 21, 71
Ritalin, 82–83
Aura, 277, 283
Author's story, 158–164
Autism, 21, 281
Autocrine hormones, 96
Autoimmune disease, 86, 152
intestinal bacteria and, 86–87
of thyroid, 58

Bahr, Richard, 78–79, 198, 256,
273
Balloon angioplasty, 74
The Bariatrician, 40–41
Bariatric medicine, 160
Barnes, Broda O., 57, 153
Basal body temperature
monitoring, 167
thyroid and, 155–157
Basophils, 95
B-cells, 94
Bedwetting, 5, 21
B-endorphins, 56
Beta-carotene, 215–216
Beta-receptors, 249
Bibliography, 309–313
Birch pollen sensitivity, 307
Blood-brain barrier, 116–117
Blood glucose, 118
Blood tests, 185–186
Blood types, 98
BMI (body mass index), 142
Body temperature. *See* Basal body
temperature
Bottled water, 223
Brady, David M., 259, 268–270

Brain, food intake and, 56
Branched-chain amino acids, 116
Breast cancer, obesity and, 35
Bronchodilators, 230
Brostoff, Jonathan, 59, 228, 234, 245, 247, 263, 265, 267, 277, 285, 310
Brushing as cellulite treatment, 252–253
Buffets, avoiding, 130
Bulimia, serotonin and, 60
Butyrate, 102–103
B vitamins, 216

Cabo-Soler, J. R., 246, 308–310
Cafarelli, David, 79, 254–255
Caffeine, 46
    cellulite prevention and, 251
Calcium supplements, 212, 216
Calorie control, 209
Cancer
    aspartame and, 140
    obesity and, 35
    yo-yo dieting and, 42
Candida protocol diet, 125
Candidiasis. *See* Yeast
Caprylic acid, 125
Carbohydrates
    candida and, 124
    emergency supply of, 181–182
    high-carbohydrate diet, 43–44
    in processed foods, 135
    serotonin levels and, 58–59
Cascade, 119
Case studies, 164–173
Celebrations, food and, 123
Cellulite, 238, 248–253
    massage, 252–253
    treatment of, 250–251
The Cellulite Solution (Dancey), 248
Centers for Disease Control and Prevention (CDC) on infertility, 10
Challenge test, 295–296, 302

Chemical Exposés (Miller & Ashford), 75
Chemoluminescence, 11–12
Children. *See also* Attention deficit disorder (ADD); Attention deficit hyperactivity disorder (ADHD)
    chronic health problems, 71
    diagnosis of, 242–243
    food intolerance in, 17–18
    migraine headaches in, 279–283
    obesity in, 30
Chlorine in water, 223–224
Chocolate, 131
Chocolate Manufacturers Association, 117–118
Cholesterol
    fatigue and, 256
    purified cholesterol, 90
Cholesterol oxides, 90–91
Chromium, 46
Chronic disease
    case study, 164–167
    meaning of, 186–188
Chronic Fatigue and Immune Dysfunction Syndrome Association of America (CFIDSAA), 266
Chronic fatigue syndrome (CFS), 5, 21, 269
    infections and, 265–266
    prevalence of, 259–260
    symptoms of, 266
Clark, William R., 88–89, 90
Classic allergic reaction, 92
Cluster headaches, 273
Co-factors, 307
Colitis, 297
Columbia/HCA Medical Center's Sports Medicine and Performance Center study, 64–66
Commercial weight-loss programs, 305
Complement system, 88

*The Complete Guide to Food Allergy
and Intolerance* (Brostoff),
265
Congestion. *See* Sinus problems
Constipation, 178
Copper, 217
Corporate Crime in the Pharmaceutical Industry (Braithwaite),
82
Cortisol, 99
Cortisone, 233
candidiasis and, 124
Coulter method, 106
Cow's milk, 236. *See also* Lactose
intolerance
Cravings, 305–306
serotonin and, 117
Cross-reactivity, 21–22, 307
Cytokines, 266

Dairy products, 100–101
*Dear America, a Concerned Doctor
Wants You to Know the Truth
about Health Reform* (Konner), 73
Deep-breathing exercises, 253
Degranulation, 95–96
Denial, 120
Depression, 21, 297
Detoxification pathway deficiency, 99–100
Dexfenfluramine, 284
Diabetes, 5, 6, 21
blood types and, 97–98
costs of caring for, 76
juvenile diabetes, 87
obesity and, 29, 35
Type 2 diabetes, 142
yo-yo dieting and, 42
Diagnosis of food intolerance, 2,
20–22
Diarrhea, 21
Diet drugs, 45–47
Diet industry, 38–42
Diets. *See also* Elimination diet;
Rotation diet

cookie-cutter diets, 204–206
high-protein diets, 2, 44–45
low-calorie diets, 39
low-fat, high-carbohydrate
diets, 144
problems with, 42–47
traditional weight loss diets, 194
for 21st century, 194–225
yo-yo dieting, 42, 112,
138–157
Digestive enzymes. *See* Enzymes
Digestive system. *See also* Gastrointestinal disorders
processed foods and, 150–151
Digitalis, 131
DNA (deoxyribonucleic acid),
102–103
microarrays, 103–104
oxygen radicals and, 89
Domino effect, 184–185
Dopamine, 56
Dose-related intolerance, 22
Driver fatigue, 162
Drug-resistant microbes, 81
Dust mites, 261
Dynophine, 56

Ear infections, 5, 21, 71
case study, 170
drug-resistant microbes, 81
Early-morning tiredness, 265
Echinacea, 218
Eczema, 21, 231–232, 238–240
percent improvement in, 245
weight loss and, 246
Edema. *See* Angioedema
Eicosanoids, 200, 206
arachidonic acid, 201
PGE-2, 200–201
Elderly people, enzyme deficiency in, 219
Elimination diet
eczema and, 247
gradually eliminating foods,
290
simple basic meals and, 289

Encyclopedia of Nutritional Supplements (Murray), 218
Endorphins, 56–57
Environmental epidemic, 74–76
Environmental physicians, 69
Enzymes
  chronic fatigue syndrome (CFS) and, 267
  in raw foods, 220
  supplements, 219–220
Ephedra, 46
Exercise. *See also* Aerobic exercise
  asthma and, 22
  cellulite prevention and, 252
  deep-breathing exercises, 253
  food sensitivities and, 181
  success of, 208

FAQs about food intolerance, 299–308
Fat blockers, 146
Fatigue, 21, 208, 254–270, 297.
  See also Chronic fatigue syndrome (CFS)
  case study, 172
  early-morning tiredness, 265
  as early warning sign, 255–259
  prevalence of, 259–262
  research on foods and, 262–265
  tension fatigue syndrome, 263–264
Fat storage
  aerobic exercise and, 299–300
  cellulite in, 249–250
  genes, 27–28
  insulin and, 119
FDA (Food and Drug Administration)
  appetite suppressants, approval of, 149
  prescription drug overuse, 83
  Recommended Dietary Allowances (RDAs), 213
  vitamins and minerals, 213
  weight-loss drugs, 48
Feast and famine cycles, 27–28

Fell, Peter, 234, 245, 263, 277, 310
Fenfluramine, 158, 284
Fen-Phen, 158, 284
Ferro, Anthony, 260, 274, 282
Fetal hemoglobin gene, 104
Fibromyalgia, 269
  case study, 167–168
  food allergy testing, 195
Filtered water, 223
Folic acid, 216
Follicle-stimulating hormone, 10
Food additives, 124
Food allergies
  and asthma, 235
  confusion with food intolerance, 6
  conventional medicine and, 189–191
  and hay fever, 235
  increased attention to, 195
  mechanisms of, 190–191
  secondary food allergies, 235
Food Allergy and Intolerance (Little), 59
Food chemicals, 75
Food intolerance
  addictive overeating and, 197–199
  confusion with food allergies, 6
  facts about, 25–26
  good news about, 196
  immune system and, 152–155
  related problems, 122
  and thyroid, 152–155
  treatment of, 77–79
  yeast overgrowth and, 129
The Food Pharmacy (Carper), 134
Food pyramid, 111, 143–144
Foods. *See also* Processed food; Safe foods
  addiction to, 177
  as drugs, 131–133
  invader foods, 179
  raw foods, 220
  simplicity of, 220–221

Four-day rotation diet, 289, 293
Foxglove, 131
Free radicals, 88–89
  cholesterol damaged by,
    90–91

Galanin, 56
Gall bladder cancer, 35
Gamma-aminobutyric acid
    (GABA), 56
Garlic, 125, 218
Gastritis, 297
Gastrointestinal disorders, 5, 6
  aspirin use and, 83
  blood types and, 98
Genetic engineering
  foods, genetically engineered,
    75
  obesity and, 51–52
Genetic polymorphism, 107
Genetic predisposition, 100–101
  food intolerance and, 306
  lactose intolerance and,
    101–102
  testing susceptibilities,
    102–107
  zinc deficiency and, 104
Gerrard, John W., 3, 78, 231, 236,
    239, 240, 280–281
Ginseng, 46, 218
Glycogen, 118–119
Gonads, 128
Gout, 42
Grains, 144–145
  refined grain products, 120
Granulocytes, 201–202
Growth hormone-releasing hor-
    mone, 56
Guilt, 120

Hanta virus, 105
Harvard Heart Letter, 55
Hay fever, 21, 227–228
  food allergies and, 235
  mast cells and, 230–231

Hayfever: The Complete Guide
    (Brostoff), 229
Hazan, Stanley, 12–14
HDL (high-density lipoprotein),
    144
Headaches, 21, 208. *See also*
    Migraine headaches
  types of, 273
Health and Medical Research
    Foundation, Texas, 65–66,
    196
Health care
  cost of, 76–77
  developments in, 69–70
  technology and, 67–69
Health insurance, 113–115
Health magazine, 257, 286
Health & Wellness Today, 73–74,
    149
Heart disease
  blood types and, 98
  food intolerance and, 12–14
  immune system and, 87
  water intake and, 224
  yo-yo dieting and, 42
Heavy metals, 124
Hein, H. O., 98
Hepatitis C, 87
Herbal remedies, 217–218
Hidden allergies, 92
High-protein diets, 2, 44–45
Hintz, Just, 227, 242–243, 271,
    274
Hippocrates, 80, 166, 298
Histamine
  asthma and, 230
  in basophils, 95
  hunger control, 56
Histograms, sample reaction,
    109
Hives, 243–244
HMOs (health maintenance
    organizations), 84
Høj, Lene, 10–11, 78, 240–241,
    261, 310–311

Hormones
    migraines and, 286
    obesity and, 56–57
Hospitals, infections from, 74
Human Nutrition, 40
Hunger
    feedback mechanisms for,
        221, 222
    signals, 55
    understanding, 147–148
Hydroxyuria, 103–104
Hyperactivity, 281. *See also* Atten-
    tion deficit hyperactivity
    disorder (ADHD)
Hyperpermeable gut, 98–99
Hypoallergenic protein formula,
    308
Hypoglycemia, lethargy and, 119
Hypothalamus, 55
Hypothyroidism, 57–58, 152–153
    new drugs for, 77
*Hypothyroidism: The Unsuspected Ill-
    ness* (Barnes & Carlton),
    57, 153

Identifying reactive foods,
    290–292
IgA antibody, 99
IgE antibodies, 93
    asthma and, 230
    RAST (radioallergosorbent
        test), 280
    testing for, 96–97
    Y shape, 94–95
Immune system
    adaptive immune system,
        91–92
    AIDS/HIV, 87
    ALCAT test and, 89–90
    allergic reaction and, 154
    atherosclerosis and, 90
    autonomy of, 179
    branches of, 91–92
    chronic fatigue syndrome
        (CFS) and, 266–267

    food intolerance and, 152–155
    herbal remedies for, 217–218
    hypothyroidism and, 58
    infertility and, 10
    innate immune system, 88,
        91–92
    intolerant foods and, 66–67
    role of, 85–91
    supplements for, 214–218
    yeast population and, 127–128
Immunoglobulin, 94
Impedance method, 105
Induction phase, 100
Infections. *See also* Yeast
    cell membranes, destruction
        of, 89
    fatigue and, 265–266
    food intolerance and, 11–12
    headaches from, 273
Infertility, 10–11
    obesity and, 35
Inflammatory bowel disease, 21
Innate immune system, 88, 91–92
Institute of Medicine obesity
    study, 29
Insulin. *See also* Diabetes
    antilipolyic effect of, 200
    aspartame and, 140–141
    carbohydrates diet and, 43–44
    effects of, 118–120
    obesity and, 56–57
    and refined grain products,
        120
    serotonin and, 116–117
    triggering rise in, 139–141
    weight loss and, 139
    yeast overgrowth and, 128
Interferon, 267
Interleukin 1 (IL1), 10
Interleukin 4 (IL4), 94
Interleukin 6 (IL6), 14
    fat cells releasing, 34
Intestinal bacteria, 86–87
Intestinal lining, 224–225
Invader foods, 179

Iron, 217
    pica, 222
Irritable bowel syndrome,
    164–167, 297

Jaconello, Paul, 199, 255–256,
    264
Japanese people, alcohol dehy-
    drogenase and, 100–101
*Journal of the American Medical
    Association (JAMA)*, 12,
    110–111, 208
Juvenile diabetes, 87

Kaats, Gilbert, 40–41, 65–66, 67,
    196–197, 246, 263–264,
    278, 311–312
Karolinska Institute, Sweden, 93
Kidney disease, 18
    obesity and cancer, 35
    water intake and, 224
Koop, C. Everett, 28
Kosher diet, 105

Lactase deficiency, 100, 306
Lactose intolerance, 100, 306
    genetics and, 101
The Lancet, 97
Larger particles of foods,
    150–151
Late-phase reaction, 95
Laxative, water as, 223
LDL (low-density lipoprotein),
    144
Leaky blood vessels, 6
Leaky gut syndrome, 98–99, 207
Legs, crossing, 252
Leptin, 51–52
Leucocytopenic index, 23
Leukocytes, 105
Leukotrienes, 96
Licorice, 46
Lipid mediators, 96
Lipofuscin, 89
Lipolysis, 200

Lipotherapie technique, 252–253
Liver and toxins, 99
Living Well with Hypothyroidism
    (Shomon), 57, 155
Low-calorie diets, 39
Low-fat, high-carbohydrate diets,
    144
Lung cancer, 236–237
Lupus, 86
Luteinizing hormone, 10
Lymphatic drainage, 252
Lymphocytes, 93–94
Lymphokines, 267

Macronutrients, 221–222
Macrophages, 10, 93
Magauran, John, 2, 78, 198
Magnesium, 216
Malaria, sickle cell trait and, 104
Malnutrition
    chronic disease and, 187
    food sensitivities and, 181–182
Mammograms, 74
Masking, 133–134
Massage, 252–253
Mast cells, 95
    asthma and, 230
    and hay fever, 230–231
    skin tests and, 96
Mastectomies, 74
Mayer, Christian, 1, 16, 232–233
Meal substitutes, 307
*A Means to an End: the Biological
    Basis of Aging* (Clark), 88
Mediators, 96
Medical technology, 67–69
Medications. *See* Over-the-
    counter (OTC) medica-
    tions; Prescription
    medications
Medscape's Web site, 143
Menstrual irregularities, 155
Messenger RNA, 104
Metabolism, hypothyroidism and,
    58

Microarrays, 103
Micronutrients, 222
Migraine headaches, 5, 6, 152,
    271–287, 297
  anatomy of, 283–284
  in children, 279–283
  classic migraine, 277
  flawed theories on, 185–187
  foods causing, 172
  serotonin and, 284, 287
Minerals, 212
Miracle diets, 37–38
Mitochondria, 270
Modern diet, 202–203
Mood swings, 4
MPOS range foods, 290–292
Mucus, increased production of,
    6
Multiple sclerosis, 86
Multivitamins, 213–214
Muscle aches, 21
Muscle loss, 41
Myeloperoxidase (MPO), 12–13

National Headache Foundation,
    272
National Institute of Diabetes, 62
Native Americans, lactase defi-
    ciency in, 101
Natural killer cells, 267
Natural Resources Defense Coun-
    cil, 75
Nausea and migraine, 277
Negative foods, 290
Neural tube defects, 35
Neurodermatitis, 242
Neuropeptides, 56
Neurotransmitters, 56
Neutrophils, 87
New England Journal of Medicine,
    51–52
Newsweek, 260
Non-steroidal anti-inflammato-
    ries (NSAIDs), 225
Norepinephrine, 56

North American Association for
    the Study of Obesity,
    113–114
Nutrition
  appetite suppressants and,
    148–149
  eating for, 211–212
  information on, 72
  stress and, 75
Nutrition Reviews Supplement,
    59–60
Nystatin, 173

Obesity, 5, 6, 8, 21, 27–61
  addictive overeating and, 197
  biochemical connection,
    54–57
  challenge test for, 296
  Columbia/HCA Medical Cen-
    ter's Sports Medicine and
    Performance Center study,
    64–66
  concerns about, 63–64
  exploring causes of, 300–301
  food intolerance and, 14–15
  hazards of, 34–35
  health costs of, 29
  health insurance and,
    113–114
  hope for, 64–66
  modern advances in weight
    loss, 50–58
  national studies, summary of,
    110–111
  questions about, 299–301
  unhappiness and, 37–38
Obesity Research, 32
Ob gene, 51
Obsessive eaters, 130–131
1+ foods, 290–292
Oral contraceptives, 124
Oregano, oil of, 125
Organically-caused headaches,
    273
Otitis media. *See* Ear infections

Ovaries, 128
Overeating, 183
  addictive overeating, 197–199
  obsessive eaters, 130–131
Over-the-counter (OTC) medications
  diet pills, 46
  for headaches, 273
Overweight. *See* Obesity

The Paleo Diet (Cordain), 86
Pancreas
  chronic fatigue syndrome
    (CFS) and, 267
  yeast overgrowth and, 128
Panic attacks, 5, 21
Pantyhose, 252
Parasites, 96
Pasula, M., 310, 312–313
Pathogens, 87
The Pathology of Drug Abuse
  (Karch), 46
Peck, Scott, 188–189
Pesticides, 261–262
PGE-2 (prostaglandin E-2),
  200–202, 284
PGI-2, 200, 284
Phagocytes, 88
Pharmaceutical companies,
  76–77
Phentermine, 125
Phospholipids, 96
Physicians, issues involving,
  73–74
Pica, 222
Pima Indians, 52–53
Pi-Sunyer, F. Xavier, 31–32, 143
Plasma cells, 94
Pleasure in eating, 123
Pneumonia, 236–237
Pollution, 75
Polymorphonuclear white blood
  cells, 201–202
Pondomin, 301
Pork, reaction to, 104–105

Pregnancy
  eczema in, 239
  food intolerance and, 152
  obesity and, 35
Prescription medications, 80–81,
  206–209
  overuse of, 82–83
  physicians and, 191–192
  for weight loss, 145–147
Processed food, 144–145
  cellulite prevention and, 251
  as dead food, 221
  enzymes and, 219
Prostaglandins, 95–96
Prostate cancer, 35
Protein
  excessive protein, 2
  high protein drinks, 307–308
Protein drinks, 307–308
Psychological trauma, 266
Psychotherapy for headaches,
  273
Purified cholesterol, 90

Questions about food intolerance, 299–308

Ragweed pollen, 96
Randolph, Theron, 257, 262,
  264–265, 273, 279
RAST (radioallergosorbent test),
  280
Ravcussin, Eric, 53
Raw foods, 220
Reactive oxygen specials, 88–89
Recommended Dietary
  Allowances (RDAs), 213
Redux, 284
Refined grain products, 120
Reintroducing foods, 163, 291,
  295, 304–305
Reperfusion, 87
Respiratory problems, 226–237
  common conditions, 230–231
  research on, 234–235

Rheumatoid arthritis, 86
Rhinitis, 171–172
    research on, 234–235
Ritalin, 82–83, 169, 171
RNA (ribonucleic acid), 104
The Road Less Traveled (Peck),
    188–189
Rotation diet, 125, 174–175,
    212–213, 218–219
    fatigue and, 256
    four-day rotation diet, 289,
    293
Rowe, Albert H., 3, 247, 262, 278

Safe foods
    mixing reactive foods with,
    303–304
    sticking to list, 293
    strategies for eating, 288–293
Salt, 252
Sandberg, Douglas, 78, 312–313
Sandweiss, Jay, 8–10, 78
Saturated fats, 120
Schimpf, Stephen, 16, 198, 233,
    248
SCIDS (severe combined
    immune deficiency), 87
Science News, 103
Scientific American, 31
Scleraderma, 86
Sears, Barry, 96, 143, 200
Secondary food allergies, 235
Selenium, 216
Self-esteem, 120
Self-medication with chocolate,
    118
Serotonin, 116–118, 177–178
    and ALCAT test, 58–60
    bulimia and, 60
    dieting and, 49–50
    hunger control, 56
    migraine headaches and, 284,
    287
    sugar and, 131
    yo-yo dieting and, 139

Serum sickness, 305–306
"Shape Up America" campaign,
    28
Sickle cell anemia, 104
Sinusitis
    case study, 228–229
    symptoms of, 231
Sinus problems, 6, 18, 21,
    164–167, 171–172, 208, 297
Skeletonized foods, 32
Skin brushing as cellulite treat-
    ment, 252–253
Skin problems, 152, 238–253, 297
    acne, 244–246
    hives, 243–244
Skin tests, 106
    for allergies, 96
Sleep deprivation, 117
Smith, Stephen, 199, 264
Smooth muscle contractions, 6
Social stigma and obesity, 35–36
Solomon, Barbara, 3–4, 198, 229,
    235, 243–244, 245–246,
    258, 262, 275–276, 287, 313
Somatic cells, 102
Spicy foods, 22
Spirulina, 218
Spreading phase, 100
Steroids
    allergens, reactions to, 292
    for asthma, 230
Stress, 4
    B vitamins and, 216
    candidiasis and, 124
    chronic fatigue syndrome
    (CFS) and, 266
    food sensitivity and, 177–179
    health issues and, 75
    leaky gut syndrome and, 98–99
    overeating and, 183
    serotonin depletion and, 117
Stuffy nose. *See* Sinus problems
Surgeon General. *See* U.S. Sur-
    geon General
Sweets, cravings for, 208

Symptoms
  of food allergies, 190
  genetic polymorphism and,
    107–108
  treatment of, 73
  of yeast overgrowth, 128

T-cells, 94
Tension fatigue syndrome,
    263–264
Tension-type headaches, 273
Testing. *See also* ALCAT test
  for airborne allergies, 92–96
  for classic allergies, 95–96
  genetic susceptibilities to
    foods, 102–107
  for hidden food allergies,
    96–101
  RAST (radioallergosorbent
    test), 280
T-helper II lymphocytes, 94
Thyroid, 57–58, 86
  body temperature and,
    155–157
  food intolerance and, 152–155
  yeast overgrowth and, 128
Thyroid.about.com, 155
Thyroiditis, 154
Thyroxin, 249
Toxic headaches, 273
Toxic intermediates, 99
Trigger foods, identifying,
    274–276
Triglycerides, 144
Tryptophan, 116–117
20th century health problems, 68
Twin studies, 306
2+ foods, 290–292
Type A blood, 97
Type AB blood, 97
Type B blood, 97
Type O blood, 97
Type 2 diabetes, 142
Tyramine, 285

University Wellness Letter, 213
Urticaria, 21, 241–242, 243–244
  percent improvement in, 245
U.S. Commerce Department, 76
U.S. Department of Agriculture
    (USDA)
  food pyramid, 111, 143–144
  obesity study, 28
U.S. News and World Report, 257
U.S. Surgeon General, 62, 114
  children, obesity in, 30
  on obesity, 28, 30
Uterine cancer, 35

Vascular headaches, 273
Vasculitis, 178
Vasodilators, 284
Vaughn, Warren T., 23, 278
Vertebra realignment, 273
Vision sensitivities, 272
Vitamin B$_6$, 216
Vitamin B$_{12}$, 216
Vitamin C, 215
Vitamin E, 215
Vitamins, 213–214
Vomiting and migraine, 277

Wall Street Journal, 77
Ward, Walter, 18, 199
Water
  body's need for, 222–224
  cellulite prevention and, 251
  filtered water, 223
  yo-yo dieting and, 141
Web sites
  Medscape's Web site, 143
  thyroid.about.com, 155
Weight cycling, 42
Weight loss
  eczema and, 246
  with Pondomin, 301
  rate of, 303
Whitaker, Julian, 73–74, 149
Whole-grain foods, 144

World Health Organization
(WHO), 33, 62
on obesity, 35

Yeast, 124–126
antibiotics and, 125
case study, 173
overgrowth, 207
progress of, 126–129

symptoms of overgrowth, 128
treating candida, 294–295
The Yeast Connection (Crook), 295
Yo-yo dieting, 42, 112, 138–157

Zinc, 216
deficiency, 104
The Zone (Sears), 96, 143, 200
Zymosan, 11

ABOUT THE AUTHORS

Rudy Rivera, M.D., practices medicine in Plano, TX and has been involved in the practice of medicine, in the fields of emergency medicine, anesthesiology and bariatrics (or, weight loss) for over thirty years. He has a special interest in weight loss because of his own problems in that area, which he overcame with the help of the Alcat test. He currently serves as Medical Director of Cell Gen Technology, LLC, in Dallas, a manufacturer of therapeutic lasers.

Roger Davis Deutsch has been involved in the research and development of the Alcat test for over 22 years. He is regarded as the world expert on food intolerance testing, weight loss and inflammatory disease. He frequently lectures on the topic world wide. He is the CEO of Cell Science Systems, Ltd., Corp. in Deerfield Beach, FL, and Alcat Europe, GmbH, in Hennigsdorf, Germany.